the
ESSENTIAL
Low Back
PROGRAM:
Relieve Pain & Restore Health

by Robin Rothenberg

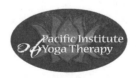

Pacific Institute
of Yoga Therapy

piyogatherapy.com

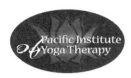

660 NW Gilman Blvd. C6
Issaquah, WA 98027

www.piyogatherapy.com

First edition 2008

A Note to the Consumer:
The information offered in this program is not intended as a substitute for the advice of physicians or other qualified health professionals. It is not intended to be prescriptive for any particular lower back condition. The consumer is advised to consult with his or her physician or health care practitioner before participating in any of the practices in this program. It is suggested that the consumer consult regularly with his or her physician with respect to any symptoms that may require further diagnosis or medical treatment. Neither the author nor publisher shall be liable or responsible for any loss, injury or damage allegedly arising from the use of any information contained in this program.

ISBN # 978-0-9802301-0-9

Library of Congress # 2008920107

Printed in the United States

Design by Elise Moyer
Illustrations by Bruce Edwards
Photography by Mary Grace Long
Music by Sasa Mlakar

ACKNOWLEDGEMENTS

It has truly taken a village to enable me to create **The Essential Low Back Program**, and I feel a deep sense of gratitude to everyone involved. First, my yoga teachers: Gary Kraftsow, for being a wonderful transmitter of the teachings of yoga, specifically in the arena of yoga therapy, and for co-authoring with me the original study protocol; Nischala Joy Devi, for her loving inspiration and constant reminder that we are Divine Beings; Karen Sherman, researcher and yogini extraordinaire, without whom there would be no Low Back Study to draw from, thank you for choosing me.

To all the Yoga Barn staff and faculty who have cheered me on, supported me, and covered for me while I've had my head in this project the past six months, you are a blessing! To all the students who allowed me to learn from the experience of their own back pain over the years, I am indebted. To Erica Slauson, who was the unseen model behind my voice, thank you. A special thanks to Arlen, Anne, Harvey, Sharon, and Taran, who kindly agreed to model and share their stories for this project.

Mary Grace, thank you for your photography skill, patience, and warmth. Lisa Farino and Rachel Bravmann thank you for your editorial expertise. Mark Newey, I appreciate your dedication and determination to get the sound 'just right' and all the tedious hours you spent at the computer. Bruce Edwards, master illustrator who supplied the artwork included, you are my hero! Sasa Mlakar, your music is the heartbeat of the CDs, I can't thank you enough! Elise Moyer, graphic designer and hand-holder really you are my guru, my guide through the dark nights of this project—thank you for your light, your laugh, your unending patience and your vision.

Jill Massengill, thanks for keeping my anatomy in check, physically and literally. Lynn Hughes thank you for supporting me in a million different ways too many to name. Patti Pitcher, word magician and friend, thank you for your willingness to step in and help, with love. Jamie Rose, thank you for your keen editing, and Ryanne for your encouragement and moral support. You two make me proud to be a mother. To Peter—thank you, thank you for never losing faith in me.

I'd like to make a special acknowledgement to Group Health Center for Health Studies in Seattle for supporting Karen and her team in bringing this valuable research to light.

TABLE OF CONTENTS

WELCOME!

About The Essential Low Back Program:

This program is based on the largest, most definitive scientific study about the use of yoga therapy for the treatment of chronic lower back pain to date. The study was funded by the National Institute of Health (NIH) and published in the [1]*Annals of Internal Medicine* in December, 2005. The 12-week program examined how participants who suffered with non-specific lower back pain responded to yoga therapy when compared with two control groups: a conventional exercise program developed by a Physical Therapist and a third group who was given a self-care book on lower back health to read.

The yoga and exercise group met once a week for 90-minute sessions and were encouraged to practice daily in the interim. The yoga participants experienced a **78% reduction in pain levels,** compared with 63% in the exercise group and 47% in the book group. The use of medication for pain management decreased most markedly among the yoga participants. In follow-up interviews, the yoga participants were the only ones who experienced continued improvement in their condition 26 weeks later. Participants in the other two groups actually experienced a worsening of symptoms a half-year later. Twice as many of the participants in the yoga classes said they would definitely recommend the yoga program to others.

The results were undeniably positive, concluding that this particular approach to yoga, known as *Viniyoga*, is a **safe and effective treatment for chronic lower back pain.** *Viniyoga* is a particularly gentle form of yoga with a strong focus on individual adaptation and breath development. *It is extremely accessible for all body types.* This study provides physicians and other western-trained medical professionals conclusive evidence for recommending *Viniyoga* and possibly other therapeutically oriented styles of yoga to their patients.

Robin Rothenberg co-authored the yoga program and worked extensively with the researchers. She taught all the classes in the original study and is now training staff for a second, larger scale NIH study, currently underway, that uses this same *Viniyoga* protocol. Now she has recreated that program, so that you have the opportunity to experience the benefits of Viniyoga through **The Essential Low Back Program** in your own home!

The CDs and accompanying booklet are *not intended to replace a medical evaluation* of your particular back condition. If you are experiencing lower back pain, please consult with a doctor before beginning this or any other yoga or exercise practice. There are some conditions, such as serious disc herniation, recent back surgery, severe sciatica, or cancer, for which this program may not be beneficial. The information in this booklet is intended to facilitate your healing through yoga. If you would like to learn more about yoga therapy or about how to connect with a yoga therapist in your area, you can visit the International Association of Yoga Therapy's website at: www.iayt.org.

[1]*Sherman KJ, Cherkin DC, Erro J, Miglioretti DL, Deyo RA. Comparing yoga, exercise, and a self-care book for chronic low back pain: a randomized, controlled trial. Ann Intern Med. 2005;143:849-56.*

HOW TO USE THIS BOOKLET

The models in this booklet are real people who have suffered from back pain and found relief through *Viniyoga*. Each practice begins with one individual's story and describes how yoga has been a vital support in regaining his or her health and well-being. At the end of each practice, you'll find some suggested reflections to help you incorporate the experience of yoga into your everyday life.

This booklet includes: **Low Back Anatomy 101**, **Introduction to Yoga in Relation to Chronic Pain**, **Breathing Basics**, **The ABC's of Yoga Posture**, and **Practice Guidelines**, in addition to five 40-60 minute yoga practices with CD companions. It is strongly suggested that you read through *all* the information in the booklet before attempting the practices. Even if you have already been practicing yoga, review is always useful and the methodology of this practice may be different than your previous approach to yoga. The practices on the CDs and in this booklet complement each other, so you can use them together or individually. Reviewing the written practices and photos prior to listening to the audio will help orient you to the kinds of movements you'll be performing. Becoming familiar with these movements through visual reference will support your skillful navigation through, and eventual mastery of this program.

The practices are designed to build on one another. The initial practice is designed to teach you basic breath and movement, cultivate your connection to your body, deepen your self-awareness, and help you relax. Relaxation is the most crucial healing tool for managing pain, developing better flexibility and muscle tone, and increasing circulation. Although the practices do become increasingly more challenging, there is no need to hurry through them. In fact, during The Low Back Study, participants stayed with this simple, initial practice for the **first three weeks** of the twelve-week program. They worked with each of the consecutive practices for two full weeks before advancing to the next. Even as they progressed, they were encouraged to refer back to this "home base" practice if they experienced a flare up or felt particularly stressed or fatigued. **Please listen to your body and progress at your own rate, supporting your body gently through its healing process.**

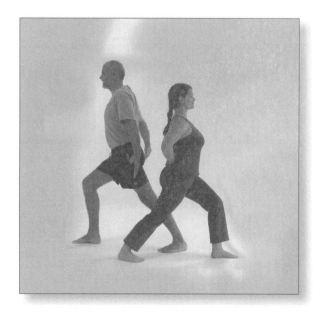

LOW BACK ANATOMY 101

The body is an amazing complex of bones, muscles, nerves, and organs that seem to communicate magically with one another to create the experience that we call healthy function. Without direction, the heart knows to beat, the lungs to breathe, and the liver to filter out toxins. For the most part, we ignore the body as long as it's doing what it "should," treating it as if it were the hired help, a servant to the mind. It's only when the body complains, as it does when injured, stressed, or left unattended for long periods of time that we bring our focus to it. Even then, we're mostly annoyed that it hurts, preventing us from enjoying the activities we love or getting a good night's rest. The body is then perceived as an obstacle to the mind's fulfillment, rather than a partner in need of some extra T.L.C..

It rarely occurs to us that the body may, in fact, be expressing the unspoken frustrations and needs of the heart. Culturally, we are attuned to physicality and most of us notice "pain" at the physical level long before we're able to acknowledge underlying mental or emotional stressors. Many clients with back pain have discovered that when they changed jobs or created better boundaries with their children, and/or spouse, their back pain dissipated. Dr. John Sarno[2] has done extensive research on this mind-body connection, specifically in relationship to chronic lower back pain. His findings show that there's no direct correlation between structural anomalies seen on an X-ray and the level of pain in a particular patient. In other words, there are people with horrific looking degenerative disc disease who are pain-free, and folks who show insignificant structural changes but can't bend over to tie their shoes. As we move into the specifics about the physical anatomy, it's important to be aware that the other levels of our consciousness are always at play. To paraphrase many great wisdom teachings: **Healing happens when the body, mind, and heart are aligned.**

As you look at **diagram 1**, note that a healthy spine is shaped in a gentle S-curve. The concavity at the lumbar and cervical regions is mirrored by the convex structures of the thoracic curve and the sacrum. These natural curvatures create a shock absorption quality and support our Homo erectus *(upright)* stance. If any of these curves are flattened out, exaggerated, or twisted due to congenital tendencies, such as scoliosis, or as a result of injury or improper usage, the spinal structure as a whole will be impacted.

Forming the base of the spine are the coccyx *(tailbone)* and the sacrum *(triangular shaped structure that establishes the center of the pelvic bowl)*, **diagram 2**. These are fused structures that allow for little movement. The five lumbar vertebrae sit above the sacrum and together form the lumbo-sacral curve, or what we commonly refer to as the "lower back". The health and balance of this curve is largely determined by the tone of the surrounding musculature. Continuing up the spine are the thoracic vertebrae, which connect to the rib cage; and the cervical vertebrae, which connect to the base of the skull.

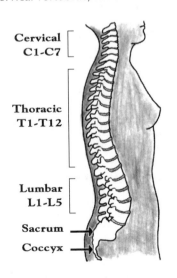

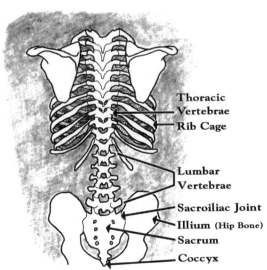

[3]diagram 1 - Spine, Side View   [3]diagram 2 - Spine, Back View

[2]John Sarno, MD, <u>Healing Back Pain</u>, Warner Books, N.Y. 1991
[3]Diagrams adapted from AVI handouts with the permission of Gary Kraftsow.

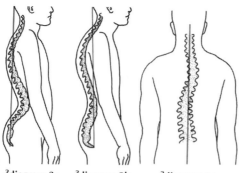

³diagram 3a
Exc. Lordosis

³diagram 3b
Exc. Kyphosis

³diagram 3c
Scoliosis

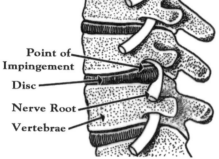

Point of Impingement
Disc
Nerve Root
Vertebrae

diagram 4 - Disc Bulge with
Nerve Impingement

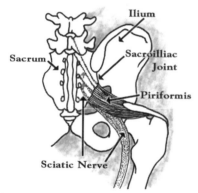

Ilium
Sacrum
Sacroilliac Joint
Piriformis
Sciatic Nerve

diagram 5 - Pelvis in Relation to Sciatic Nerve
Posterior View

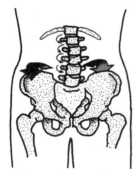

diagram 6 - Sacro-iliac
(S.I.) Joint Misalignment

The most common structural anomalies that directly impact the spine are lordosis (excessive lumbar curvature), and kyphosis (excessive upper back curvature), **diagram 3a and b.** Some people have an excessively flattened lower or upper back, and this too can be problematic. Scoliosis, or curvature of the spine, **diagram 3c** is a unique and complex variable that we will not be addressing specifically in this booklet. However, the practices in this program will be useful for most people with mild scoliosis. You can check with your doctor if you are concerned about having any of these conditions.

The intervertebral discs sit between the bony structure of the vertebrae creating a cushioning effect. In cases of spinal degeneration or herniation, the gel-like disc material either dries up or pushes out from the edge of the vertebral column and can put pressure on the spinal nerves **diagram 4.** Both of these conditions can lead to varying degrees of pain and discomfort. Because of the complex nerve plexus that runs through the lumbo-sacral area *(particularly the sciatic nerve and it's off-shoots)* **diagram 5**, pin-pointing the exact source of pain in this region, makes a specific diagnosis difficult to determine. Symptoms can be alleviated by releasing pressure on the nerves through proper postural alignment and re-organization of the spinal musculature through conscious movement like yoga.

Where the sacrum and the illium *(pelvic bones)* meet, they form the sacro-iliac *(S.I.)* joint **diagram 5**. This joint, unlike most joints in the body is not intended to move the body. Instead, its primary function is stabilization. Excessive torsion or rotation of the S.I. joint can sprain the ligaments that hold the bones in place **diagram 6**. A sprained S.I. joint becomes inflamed, swollen, and sore in much the way a sprained ankle does. Unfortunately, it's hard to put a splint on the pelvis to immobilize it so it can heal. Every twist, turn, rotation, and flexion of the spine can possibly re-inflame the area. Repetitive injury to this region can permanently overstretch the S.I. ligaments and destabilize the pelvis. In this case, building and maintaining strength in the musculature that surrounds the sacrum is a critical part of the healing process and a primary focus for our work in therapeutic yoga.

³*Diagrams adapted from AVI handouts with the permission of Gary Kraftsow.*

All of the bony structures of the spine are held in place by soft tissue: muscles, tendons, ligaments, and fascia. Tendons attach muscle to muscle and muscle to bone. Ligaments attach bone to bone. Both tendons and ligaments are more fibrous *(thicker)* and have less blood circulating through them than muscles. This is why it's harder to heal tendon and ligament damage than injured muscle. Fascia is the saran-wrap-like sheath that surrounds the other soft tissue structures and connects one structure to the other. When the soft tissue is healthy, it has resilient tone, free range of movement and good circulation. However, in the case of injury, strain, or chronic tension, these structures may be functionally compromised, locked in a state of contraction, or stuck together by scar tissue. When this occurs movement is restricted and blood flow is impeded which can potentially lead to pain.

In the case of lower back pain, it is rare that one particular muscle is the culprit. Our muscles, much like ourselves, function in relationship with others. These relationships can either support integrity and balance or lead to dysfunction. For instance, if a muscle on the front of the body is particularly tight, it will pull the pelvis forward and lead to compression on the back side, subsequently, on the discs in the lumbar region. *(like the iliopsoas, reference pg. 10,* **diagram 14 & 15***)* If the right side of a paired muscle group is tighter than the left, it can pull the pelvis to the right and create torsion on the sacroiliac joint. **diagram 7**. These interconnected relationships between muscles are aptly called agonist/antagonist. They can literally set off a domino effect of reactivity throughout the low back and pelvic girdle.

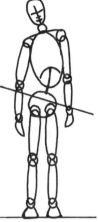

diagram 7
Pelvic Torsion

The primary function of the more exterior muscles, *(those closer to the surface)* is to mobilize or move the body. Muscles like the hamstrings and quadriceps, for instance, act as our primary ambulatory muscles. The more intrinsic layers of muscle *(closer to the bone)*, such as the transversus abdominus and multifidus *(see Accessing Your Inner Core, pg. 12)*, are intended to stabilize or hold the bones in place. When our stabilizers are not in good shape, our mobilizers end up multi-tasking, trying to hold us together and move us at the same time. The net result is chronically tight muscles that don't move well and are unable to support us in staying erect. In other words, the weak stays weak, the tight stays tight. This almost always translates directly into chronic pain.

WHY YOGA WORKS

Yoga works from the inside out. By slowing movement down, deepening the breath, and consciously using the breath to link movement with awareness, we begin to dismantle many of the tightly woven patterns of contraction that created the imbalance in the first place. Slow movement allows us to access the deeper, more intrinsic muscles and wake them up so they can begin to do the job of stabilization again. Gentle stretching combined with contraction in sequence, loosens the layers of tension held in the surface muscles and encourages greater circulation to those areas. Utilizing combinations of asymmetrical and symmetrical postures shed light on the subtle right/ left imbalances which have accrued over time. Gradually, we begin to re-calibrate these muscular warps and establish a new sense of balance, one that supports optimum health and well-being.

MUSCLES of the LOW BACK and PELVIS and HOW THEY WORK

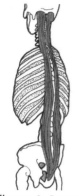

diagram 8 - Erectors

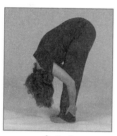

photo 1
Standing Forward Bend

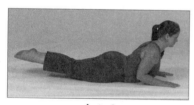

photo 2
Cobra Pose with Leg Lifts

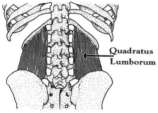

diagram 9
Posterior View

Quadratus
Lumborum

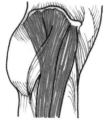

diagram 10
Gluteus Muscles

There are three primary sets of muscles that play a starring role in the balance of the pelvis and low back. On the back side are the erectors, the quadratus lumborum, the glutes, and the hamstrings. On the inside core are the pelvic floor, the transversus abdominus, the multifidi and the illio-psoas (pronounced, illio-so-as). In addition to these, the adductors, the abductors (inner and outer thigh muscles), and hip rotators are important for stabilizing the pelvic girdle and releasing pressure off the sciatic nerve.

On The Backside:

THE ERECTORS diagram 8 - The erectors are the muscles that run lengthwise along the spinal column. They do exactly what their name implies – hold us erect. They can be locked long *(that is held habitually in an overstretched position, as with chronic slump)* or locked short *(as in the case of lumber lordosis - excessive low-back arch)*. Ideally, the erectors are strong and well-supported by the deep core muscles *(the transversus abdominus and the mutifidus)*, and the skeletal bones of the legs, pelvis and spine, providing good postural alignment. Forward bends stretch the erectors, **photo 1** and back bends like the **Cobra Variations, photo 2** strengthen them.

QUADRATUS LUMBORUM diagram 9 - The quadratus spans either side of the spine across the lumbar region, below the rib-cage, and connect to the sacrum at the bottom. Most often when people put their hands to the small of the back on the sides and complain, "Oy, my back hurts!," their hands are pressing into the quadratus. The quadratus is like the sentry for the low back. With any sign of strain or torsion in the lumbo-sacral region, the quadratus lock down in a splinting action to keep further damage from happening. The challenge with long-term back problems is that often quadratus on one or both sides has been on guard for so long, it has literally forgotten how to relax, which impedes circulation and circumvents healing. Side Bends and twists in particular, help stretch the quadratus as do forward bends like *The Wheel.

*See pg. 24 for a full description of **The Essential Low Back Program's** version of **The Wheel.**

GLUTEUS MUSCLES diagram 10 - The glutes or "butt" muscles, in conjunction with the hamstring and quadriceps *(back and front thigh muscles)*, are responsible for the mobility and stability of our pelvis. Since their primary purpose in life is to "walk us," they are happiest when well-used. Sitting or standing for extended periods of time actually tires them out. When weakened from disuse, they lose their capacity to provide support for the pelvis, a set up for potential problems in the hips, sacrum, and lower back. If excessively tight, they can put pressure on the sciatic nerve, creating a proverbial pain in the a--.

Correction

The second paragraph on page 3 should read:

The yoga and exercise group met once a week for 90-minute sessions and were encouraged to practice daily in the interim. Seventy-eight percent of the yoga participants experienced a significant reduction in pain levels, as compared with 63% in the exercise group and 47% in the book group. Those who participated in the yoga group decreased their use of medication for pain management more significantly than those in other treatment programs. In follow-up interviews, the yoga participants were also the only ones to report that they experienced continued improvement in their condition 26 weeks after the end of the yoga program. Participants in the other two groups reported that they actually experienced a worsening of their symptoms six months later. Of those who participated in the programs, those who used yoga were twice as likely as other participants to recommend their treatment method to others suffering low back pain.

For information on the research supporting the validity and importance of viniyoga in relieving low back pain, see www.piyogatherapy.com.

THE HAMSTRINGS diagram 11 - There are actually three hamstring muscles, one that sits towards the outer thigh, one more to the inside line, and one that runs down the center of the back of the upper leg. The hamstrings originate at the sit-bones *(just under the flesh of the buttocks)* and run down the thigh to the knee, where they morph into the calf muscles, which, at the juncture of the ankle become the Achilles heel. In other words, the whole back side of the lower body from the bottom of the foot *(plantar fascia)*, all the way up is connected. When any part of the back of the body is excessively tight, it inhibits movement on all parts. This is the result of the fascia or connective tissue that literally holds it all together. Tightness in the hamstrings is very common among those who sit for a living or engage in recreational sports like running or biking, especially if they don't stretch regularly. This can create undue stress on the lower back by pulling the pelvic girdle down and restricting its ability to rotate easily, thus reducing the healthy curvature of the lumbar spine.

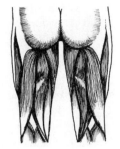

diagram 11
Hamstrings

Fun Experiment: To demonstrate this connectivity, from a standing position, try bending forward gently and feel the tightness on the back of the legs. Then stand back up and roll your right foot for 3-4 minutes over a tennis ball. Then, bend forward again. Notice the difference. Of course, you'll need to balance yourself by rolling your left foot on the ball for an equal length of time. For those with chronic foot pain, like plantar fasciitis, this exercise can be very useful for reducing pain and inflammation not just in the feet, but also in the lower back!

On The Inside:

THE PELVIC FLOOR diagram 12 - These muscles form a diamond-shaped sling, attaching from the tail bone to the pubic bone. Many women may be familiar with these muscles through 'Kegel' exercises, which are often prescribed to tone the pelvic floor after giving birth. These muscles offer a foundation of support for the whole pelvic girdle. Maintaining healthy tone in the pelvic floor benefits not only the musculoskeletal structure, but is also beneficial for the urinary tract, the prostate, and the reproductive organs. For more specifics on how to activate the pelvic floor; (see *Accessing the Inner Core, pg. 12).*

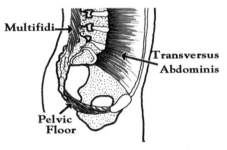

diagram 12 - Pelvic Floor, Transversus
Abdominis, Multifidi

TRANSVERSUS ABDOMINIS diagram 12 - The Transversus is the deepest layer of abdominal muscle. It extends from the pubic bone to the navel. Toning the transversus is not about creating a set of six-pack abs. More importantly, it is critical for maintaining stability in the lower back. Throughout this program, we refer to the action of transversus as engaging the lower abdominals. When this contraction is combined with the engagement of the multifidus, the pelvic floor, and diaphragm, all together, they create the Inner Core; (see *Accessing the Inner Core pg. 12).*

MULTIFIDUS diagram 12 - The multifidi are tiny, zipper-like muscles that connect each vertebra to the next, from the base of the lumbar spine, all the way up to the skull. They are deep-set muscles which lie underneath the erectors and are an integral part of the "Inner Core." They are a bit challenging to access, and work best in tandem with the transversus abdominus and the pelvic floor (see *Accessing the Inner Core, pg. 12).* When the multifidi are strong, they provide deep stabilization for the lumbo-sacral spine and allow the erectors and other more superficial muscles of the back to relax.

ILIO-PSOAS *(pronounced il-i-o-so-as)* **diagram 13** - The iliacus and psoas together form the ilio-psoas, which are major players in maintaining healthy pelvic lumbar movement. The psoas runs from the top of the lumbar *(T12-L1)* through the pelvis, where it merges with the iliacus and inserts into the inner thigh. These muscles are responsible for hip flexion and hip extension. When the psoas is locked short **diagram 14** *(as it is in many people)*, it pulls the whole pelvis forward, creating lordosis (excessive lumbar curve; compare to **diagram 15**). When the psoas is weak *(also very common)*, it does not provide adequate support for the low back and pelvis. More often than not, with sacro-iliac *(S.I.)* misalignment and instability, one side of the psoas is hyper-contracted, creating torsion and great discomfort around the sacrum. *(refer back to pg. 6 for a description of pelvic misalignment).*

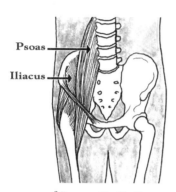

Psoas

Iliacus

[3]diagram 13 - Ilio-Psoas
Front View

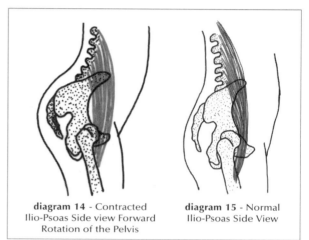

diagram 14 - Contracted
Ilio-Psoas Side view Forward
Rotation of the Pelvis

diagram 15 - Normal
Ilio-Psoas Side View

In The Pelvic Girdle:

THE ADDUCTORS AND ABDUCTORS diagram 16 -
These are the muscles of the inner and outer thighs, which provide foundational support for our postural alignment. The adductors *(inner thigh muscles)* are the top end of a fascial line that begins at the arch of the foot and runs up the inside line of the leg ending at the pelvic floor. This line of muscles needs to be well-toned and flexible to support balance and agility in movement. Pronation of the feet *(collapsed arches)* or habitually standing and sitting with the feet and hips "ducked out" in a ballerina kind of position, cause this inner foundation to sag, and weakens the whole pelvic girdle. **Mountain Pose** awareness, as we practice in yoga, helps to break this pattern and tone the adductors. Hip stretches like the **Butterfly** and **Leg Extensions** with legs straddled help stretch and tone the adductors. Like-wise, lack of tone or excessive tightness in the abductors on the outer thigh can play a significant role in chronic sacrum instability and hip pain. These muscles *(which connect to the iliotibial band, a fibrous, non-vascular band of fascia intended for stabilization as we walk)*, can also be both tight and weak from lack of use. Postures like the **Side-Hip Strengtheners** and **Hip Circles** actively work the abductors and can help alleviate sciatic nerve inflammation in the hip and upper leg.

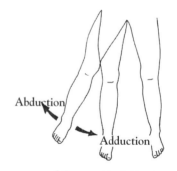

Abduction

Adduction

[3]diagram 16 - Adduction
and Abduction

[3]Diagrams adapted from AVI handouts with the permission of Gary Kraftsow.

The Pelvic Stabilizers:

HIP ROTATORS diagram 17 - The rotator muscles of the hips do exactly what their name implies. They are responsible for moving the ball of the femur *(thigh bone)* in the socket of the pelvis. The rotator muscles are small and mighty. They hold the largest joint in the body together *(the hip joint)*, and enable us as bi-pedal beings to move in many different directions. Unfortunately, unless we are dancers, gymnasts, soccer players, or yogis, we rarely have occasion to rotate our hips out or in, or even extend them, as in a lunge. We mostly hinge at the hips, flexing them as in sitting down, standing up, and walking forward. Under-utilization of the rotators makes them tight and weak. This can lead not only to sore, achy hips and an unstable pelvis, it can also create impingement of the sciatic nerve, which weaves through these muscle layers *(particularly the piriformis muscle)*, leading to sciatica-like symptoms. Asymmetrical tightness can also pull on the sacro-iliac joint and create misalignment of the pelvic girdle. Any movement that increases external and internal hip rotation, such as the poses previously mentioned as well as **Cobra Swimmer's Variation** and **Leg Cradle**, will help to exercise the hip rotators.

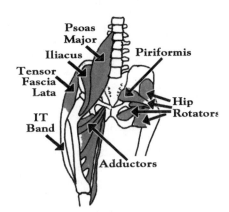

diagram 17 - Hip Rotators

Since everything in the body is connected to everything else, *("The thigh bone's connected to the shin bone")*, **diagram 18** there are many other muscles and structural factors that can impact the lower back. This brief anatomy lesson was not intended to be comprehensive, but rather to educate you about some of the more prominent muscle groups that support optimum low back health. These are the very muscle groups that we'll be targeting in **The Essential Low Back Program.**

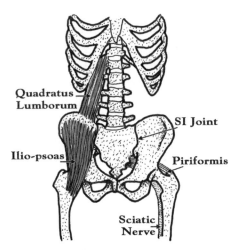

diagram 18 - Pelvic Girdle Front View

ACCESSING YOUR INNER CORE

The Players diagram 19:

The **DIAPHRAGM** is your primary breathing muscle and is located underneath the rib cage. It is a dome-like sheath of muscle which divides the thoracic and abdominal cavities. This" breathing muscle" is the "roof" of the Inner Core. See page 15, **diagram 20**.

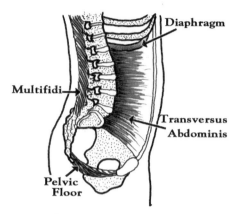

diagram 19 - The Inner Core

The **PELVIC FLOOR** is a sling of muscles that connect the pubic bone to the anal sphincter. It is the "floor" of the Inner Core muscles.

The **TRANSVERSUS ABDOMINUS**, the deepest layer of the abdominal muscles, is located between the prominent bony landmarks on the front of the pelvis. The transversus extends from the pubic bone to the navel and is referred to as the lower abdominals. It is the "front" of the Inner Core muscles. Think of them as the "shhhhh muscles," because if you "shhhh" and squeeze in and up from the lower belly, you'll feel them contract and engage.

The **LUMBAR MULTIFIDI** are the smallest and deepest layer of the back muscles that link each vertebra of the spine with the next. They form the "back" of the Inner Core and provide direct lumbar *(lower back)* vertebral stabilization. Think of them as the "zipper muscles," as they create a ladder-like zipper that runs up the spine.

The following exercises are useful for developing awareness of the Inner Core muscles. They can be used as independent isolation exercises or combined for stronger effect. Once this basic level of muscular isolation is mastered, these exercises can be incorporated into other activities including: lifting, bending, sitting, walking, yoga and other exercises or activities. With the engagement of the Inner Core, you're basically teaching your body to stabilize correctly from the inside out.

1. **DIAPHRAGMATIC BREATHING**: Begin by focusing on your breathing, observing where you feel your inhale move your rib cage. Next, try to change the focus of your breathing and expand your rib cage evenly in all directions like you are blowing up a balloon. The expansion should be even, front to back, top to bottom, including both sides. Practice this deep diaphragmatic breathing frequently throughout your day for mini stress-relief; it could be as simple as one breath, but would be more beneficial to practice 8-12 breaths at a time. This is the primary inhalation technique used in yoga breathing.

2. **PELVIC FLOOR**: This isolation exercise uses the same muscles as if you were stopping your pee in midstream. *(If you are having trouble isolating these muscles, practice this the next time you use the restroom. However, do not stop your flow as a regular practice, as it is not good for your urinary system.)*

    • To contract both the superficial and the deep pelvic floor, visualize the muscles that line the bottom of the pelvis as a drawstring. Cinch them in and draw them together and up.

    • Try not to contract the rectal portion of the pelvic floor, isolate the front only. This takes some practice. Initially, you may feel the anal sphincter and the glutes engage. Begin to release them while maintaining muscular contraction on the front side of the pelvic floor.

2. PELVIC FLOOR *continued:*

- Another helpful way to isolate these muscles is to visualize an elastic cord between your feet extending up toward the belly button. Pull up from the floor to your belly button.

- Hold for 10 seconds several times during the course of the day.

3. TRANSVERSUS ABDOMINUS: *(The "shhhhh muscles")* Slowly and gently pull your lower abdomen inward. Imagine trying to "zip-up" a slightly too-tight pair of pants.

- The movement should be a pulling in of the deep muscles, not a bulging out of the more superficial ones.

- Imagine an elastic cord running between the two prominent bony points on the front of the pelvis. Squeeze in as if cinching that cord.

- Placing your hands on your lower abdominals may help you access transversus, as you feel a subtle tensing of the muscle under your fingertips.

- Hold this action for 10 seconds several times each day.

4. THE LUMBAR MULTIFIDI: *(The zipper muscles")* To activate these tiny muscles, create a forward tilt in the pelvis *(tailbone out, back slightly arched)* and think of hugging your spine 360 degrees, or narrowing the sides of the body in towards center. This contraction should be isometric, meaning you can feel the tensing of the muscles, but there's no discernible movement.

- Another image is to think about an elastic cord running between the "dimples" in your lower back. Think about tightening the cord between your dimples, pulling them closer together.

- Hold this position for 10 seconds several times during the course of the day.

These isolation exercises can be done individually or as a group. To activate the whole Inner Core: Take a deep breath from your diaphragm, allowing your ribs to expand to the front, back and sides. Allow the air to exhale naturally. Before you take another breath, slowly and gently contract your Inner Core *(pelvic floor, "shhhh muscles"/transversus abdominus, then the zipper muscles/lumbar multifidus).* Inhale and release the contraction. Repeat. The feeling of having the whole Inner Core engaged should feel like you've created an inner girdle that deeply supports your lower spine. Practice taking and releasing the Inner Core several times, then begin to sustain the engagement for several breaths at a time. Build gradually, resuming normal diaphragmatic breathing while maintaining contraction of your Inner Core. Hold for up to 6 breaths.

Once you are familiar with the postures in this program, you can begin to integrate core work into your practice. The postures that are most useful for working the Inner Core are the extension postures, like **Seated** and **Standing Mountain Pose**, **Butterfly Pose** and back-bending postures like the **Cobra Variations**, **Warrior** and **Bridge**. The pelvic floor and transversus are also important to engage during **Forward Bends**, **Twists**, and **Lateral Bends**, as they offer additional support to the low back.

INTRODUCTION TO YOGA IN RELATION TO CHRONIC PAIN

Yoga is an ancient science of mind and body that developed out of the Indus valley in India some 5,000 years ago. The original intent of the practices and teachings of yoga was to help us actualize our potential and free us from suffering. The teachings offer a wide array of techniques, with the recognition that suffering can occur on the physical, psychological, and spiritual realms and is often a mix of all of the above.

Unfortunately, in the west, contemporary yoga has extrapolated these complex and meditative practices of yoga to fit our physical culture. Focusing principally on mastery of the body, as can be observed in photos of yogis performing contortionist postures, mainstream yoga has become more of a sport than a serious discipline designed for personal transformation, as it was originally intended.

In reality, the ancient yogis were far more interested in where we place our attention than whether we can place our leg behind our head. By observing the nature of their own minds, they concluded that the human experience *(whether painful or not painful)* was entirely based on perception. Our perception is largely colored by our mood, and our mood is created primarily by the choices we make throughout our day. Following this logic, how we feel five minutes from now or tomorrow will have much to do with the choice we are making in this very moment. For instance, if we sit at a computer terminal all day, commute for 45 minutes each way, eat fast food, and take little time for exercise, self-reflection, relationships, and fun, we can hardly expect to feel good.

> Our body, mind, and spirit will respond to the "fuel" we put into our proverbial tank. According to yoga, we're not just what we eat, but the sum total of what we eat, speak, think, and do. In essence, everything matters. However, most of us don't bother to pay attention to this equation until something goes wrong.

Pain is usually the indicator we use for "something going wrong." Rather than seeing pain as a negative, think of it metaphorically as the body's way of getting our attention, like the smoke detector in your home. It's there to alert you of a problem and to call you to take action. If you deactivate the detector because you find the noise annoying, by the time you realize there's a problem you could be engulfed in a three-alarm fire. In the same way, if we anesthetize our pain, tune it out, or push past it, we're ignoring our innate and ingenious alarm system from doing what it's intended to do: **Alert us to take action!**

When we're caught in the cycle of chronic pain, flitting from doctor appointment to therapist office, it's hard to imagine that there's anything more we could be doing to help ourselves. *Relax.* In fact, slowing down and learning to relax are some of the best coping skills for stopping the insidious repetition of dysfunctional and painful patterns in our lives. Breathing practices, combined with simple movements done slowly, help our nervous system to unwind and teach us how to literally let go of tension.

This is one of the magical elements of yoga. When we slow down, we create space. In that space, we can begin to see more clearly what's actually happening: how we chronically tighten our shoulders, or brace our back by tensing our buttocks, or feed ourselves negative messages that are self-limiting and destructive.

We're hard-wired to form habits and routines, whether they support us in health or not. However, when we learn to activate the pause button, we can create healing opportunities that allow us to do things differently than the way we've done them in the past. This is a critical piece of the process. Doing things differently may mean getting a new mattress *(one that better supports the back)*, talking through some long-harbored resentment with your partner, doing a 30-minute yoga practice, or taking a walk in nature. Sometimes it's as simple as taking a few deep conscious breaths before responding to the co-worker you find particularly irritating.

One of the interesting discoveries the yogis made is that the more healing opportunities we create, the healthier and more vibrant we feel. Each time we set in motion a new way of perceiving and responding to our world and ourselves, we strengthen our capacity to cope with the stressors of life with more agility and ease. Once we learn the mechanism for shifting out of the habitual and into the new in one area of our lives, we can transfer that experience to other arenas as well. In **The Essential Low Back Program**, we're focusing on developing optimum lower back health, but the basic principles of yoga can be applied to optimizing any aspect of your life.

BREATHING BASICS

The respiratory system is one of the most unique and remarkable features of our bodies. Respiration is controlled by the autonomic nervous system, which is to say, it functions without us needing to remind it to do its job. However, unlike some of the other automatic systems in our body *(like the circulatory system)*, we can put respiration into manual overdrive. I've not met anyone who can shift the direction of the blood flow in her body by simply thinking about it, but all of us can shift our breathing pattern with a little thought and practice. Instinctively, we know this. When we encounter someone who has suffered a trauma of some sort and is panicky, we advise him or her to "Take a deep breath." Deep breathing has long been equated with a calmer, more relaxed state of mind. However, few of us have ever been instructed in how to breathe effectively.

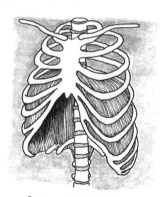

[3]**diagram 20** - Diaphragm

As we inhale efficiently, the diaphragm *(a thin sheath of muscle which sits under the rib cage)* **diagram 20**, contracts and moves down. This creates a vacuum effect, drawing air into the lungs. With exhalation, the diaphragm relaxes and moves back up under the ribs, helping to push the air out of the body, **diagram 21**. In addition to the diaphragm, the other primary breathing muscles are the intercostals, which weave between the ribs and wrap around the sides of the body. Like any other set of muscles, the respiratory muscles can be strong and flexible, or tight and weak. Deep yoga breathing or **Pranayama**, helps develop our respiratory capacity by exercising our primary breathing muscles, as well as secondary breathing muscles like the abdominals, to make the breathing experience more dynamic.

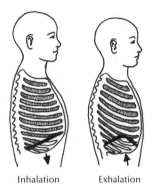

Inhalation   Exhalation

[3]**diagram 21** - Action of the Diaphragm in Healthy Respiration

[3]*Diagrams adapted from AVI handouts with the permission of Gary Kraftsow.*

> Increased respiratory capacity inspires the relaxation response, strengthens the immune and digestive systems, alleviates anxiety, and promotes a good night's sleep.

How we breathe can literally dictate how we feel. For instance, shallow chest breathing triggers the "fight-or-flight" phenomenon. If the diaphragm doesn't move freely as we breathe, it creates an environment that breeds chronic tension by blocking the lung's ability to expand fully. This sets up an internal message loop that our system is under duress. When the body and mind are receiving stress messages, everything contracts. Chronic subliminal contractions *(the kind we do unconsciously)* often lead to pain. If you carry tension in your neck, this could lead to headaches. If you carry stress in your back, this could create back pain.

The good news is that by developing healthier breathing habits we can reduce or even eliminate this pattern of chronically held tension. The breath provides a perfect conduit for the re-patterning process mentioned earlier. Since we're all habituated to breathe in a particular way *(multiplied by X number of breaths per minute, multiplied by the hours, days, and years of our lives)*, our breath is a virtual playground for us to practice creating healing opportunities. You'll find that each of the practices in **The Essential Low Back Program** begins and ends with deep yoga breathing and that all the movements are coordinated with the breath. The emphasis on the breath is intentional to teach you a powerful tool for calming your own nervous system and unwinding yourself out of pain.

THE ABC'S OF YOGA POSTURE

There are five directions in which the spine can move: **Spinal Extension, Forward Bending, Back Bending, Lateral Bending** and **Twisting**. Ideally, we experience a sense of freedom without discomfort in all of them.

The first direction is **Spinal Extension**, which is an upward, intervertebral lift, moving us out of our habitual slump into what's commonly known as "good posture." In yoga terms, we call this **Mountain Pose, photos 3** and **4**, and it is considered the basis for all other yoga postures. **Mountain Pose** requires lots of support from those little intrinsic muscles as well as a keen awareness of how we hold our body upright in space. Developing the capacity to sustain a Mountain Pose awareness throughout our daily life takes practice and constant reinforcement. **diagram 22**.

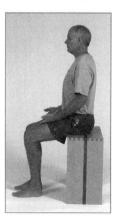

photo 3 - Mtn. Pose Sitting

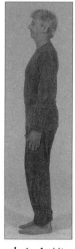

photo 4 - Mtn. Pose Standing

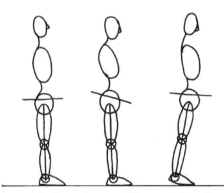

Proper Mtn. Pose Alignment   Improper Alignment of Mtn. Pose

diagram - 22

The second direction of movement is **Forward Bending**, which stretches the back of the body. **Forward Bends** can be done standing, **photo 5**, kneeling, **photo 6**, sitting, or lying on the back. They can be symmetrical or asymmetrical **photo 7**. However, the primary intention of the forward bend movement is to stretch the back, which requires forward flexion or rotation of the pelvic girdle. Most of our lives are spent in this kind of forward flexion, whether we're sitting at a computer table, driving in our car, or slumped on the couch, watching T.V. **diagram 23**. Our typical, unconscious seated posture doesn't provide much positive stretch or active support for the back. Most forward bends in the world of yoga require a **Mtn. Pose** awareness of spinal extension in order to achieve their full benefit, **photo 8.**

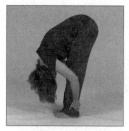

photo 5 - Symmetrical Forward Bend

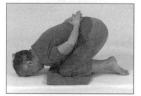

photo 6 - Kneeling Forward Bend

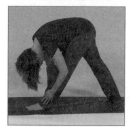

photo 7- Asymmetrical Forward Bend

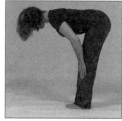

photo 8 - Forward Bend with Mtn. Pose Extension

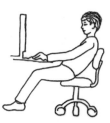

diagram 23
Typical Seated Slump

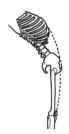

diagram 24
Hyper-extension/ Back Bending

The third direction is **Back Bending**, which requires hyper-extension *(beyond Mtn. Pose extension)* **diagram 24** of the spine and stretches the front of the body. Unlike **Extension** and **Forward Bending**, most of us do not engage in back bending movements unless we attend a yoga or dance class, or are involved in a physical therapy program. Because we spend so much time forward bending *(unconsciously)*, back bends provide the body with an antidote, creating more length along the front of the body **photo 9**. If done correctly, back bending will also strengthen the back of the body, **photo 10** rectifying weakened and underdeveloped muscles that our sedentary lifestyle tends to promote.

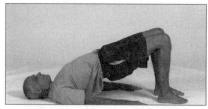

photo 9 - Bridge Pose, Back Bending

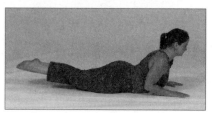

photo 10 - Cobra Pose with Leg Lifts, Back Bending

*Forward and Backward Rotation of the pelvis are the two primary ways the pelvic girdle is intended to move. Ease of movement in the pelvis is key to lumbo-sacral health. **The Essential Low Back Program** provides lots of experiential practice of these two movements with each and every repetition of **The Wheel Pose**. Coming to understand this movement in your own body will greatly aid your healing process. photos 11 and 12.*

The fourth direction is **Lateral Bending, photo 13,** which opens up the sides of the body and stretches into the shoulders, upper back and arms. When the sides are tight, they create undue stress that can pull us out of alignment. Learning to stretch into the sides of the body is an important part of any good yoga program. **Side bends** help to stretch the intercostal muscles and greatly aid in the development of respiratory capacity. The challenge in side-bending is to avoid torsion or twisting in the pelvis, by actively engaging the lower abdominals and stabilizing the lumbo-sacral area.

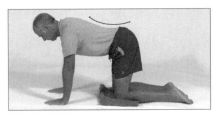

photo 11 - Forward Rotation with
Spinal Extension (Back Bend)

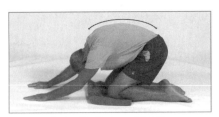

photo 12 - Backward Rotation
with Spinal Flexion (Forward Bend)

The fifth direction is **Spinal Twisting, photo 14.** We do not live symmetrically in our bodies. Certain jobs require repetitive movements that mold us into a torqued position. I had one client who had been a dentist for 50 years. His body had literally contorted to the shape of his position at the dental chair, twisting over his patients to access their mouths. Conscious twisting poses helped to unravel his torsion and re-establish symmetry, eventually alleviating a good deal of his back pain. Twisting postures can also help to free us up to safely engage in recreational activities such as tennis, golf, or dancing.

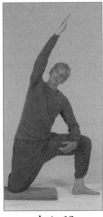

photo 13
Lateral Bend

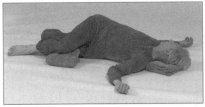

photo 14 - Lying (Spinal) Twist

Sequencing Basics:

How these postures are combined with one another will have a huge impact on your yoga experience. Generally, beginning and ending with a symmetrical forward bend is a good idea. This stretches the spinal muscles evenly from the start, and realigns them at the finish. **Back bends**, **Laterals** and **Twists** all create some level of contraction of the back muscles *(either symmetrically or asymmetrically)*. Interspersing symmetrical **Forward bends** in between the other directions of movement makes logical sense to release back tension that may have been created along the way. Therefore in good yoga sequencing we use **Forward bends** as the hub to alleviate any potential imbalance created by the other postures. **diagram 25**.

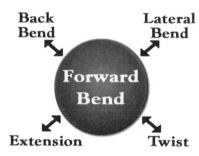

diagram 25 - Sequencing Principals

There isn't one supreme posture that will 'fix' your back. *What makes the difference is the relationship between the postures and how they are used to transform the neuro-muscular patterns of your movements.*

The most important thing for you to remember is that each sequence in **The Essential Low Back Program** *has been carefully designed to support you safely through your practice.*

> Extrapolating bits and pieces from one practice to another or performing the poses out of order puts you at risk of injury.

Sample Practice Demonstrating Sequencing Principles

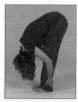
1. Forward Bend

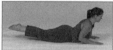
2. Back bend

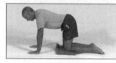
3a. Back bend

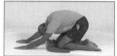
3b. Forward Bend

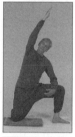
4. Lateral Bend

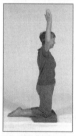
5a. Extension *(preparation for Forward Bend)*

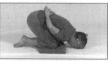
5b. Forward Bend

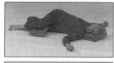
6. Twist

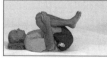
7a. Forward Bend

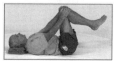
7b. Forward Bend

PRACTICE GUIDELINES

If you are working on your own, please use these practices in the order in which they are presented. If you are working with a trained yoga teacher or therapist, she may advise you to make particular adaptations for your condition, in which case you should follow your teacher's suggestions. You'll notice that there are various adaptations offered in the booklet *(such as sitting on a chair instead of kneeling for those with knee problems)*. Please use the variations that are appropriate for you. They are not lesser postures, rather, they are ways of accessing the same muscle groups safely, without putting stress on other vulnerable areas.

As with any rehabilitation process, the results will correspond to how consistent you are with your practice. Daily practice is recommended, choosing the time of day that will allow you to fully relax and enjoy the experience. If you're an early morning person, starting your day with practice might make sense. If you're not, don't attempt to impose a schedule that will most likely become an obstacle to getting to your mat. Morning, early evening, or before bed are all wonderful times of day for yoga. Choose the one that matches your energy and the flow of your day so that this practice will enhance your lifestyle rather than conflict with it. Practicing on an empty, or mostly empty, stomach is advised, so evening practice should be spaced a few hours after dinner. Sometimes it's helpful to keep a practice journal so you can track your healing process week to week.

When working with your breath, the key is to stay relaxed. If you become aware that you are grasping for or struggling with your breath, pause and resume your natural inhalation and exhalation. Release tension in your body and then gradually begin to work with the yoga breathing as you feel comfortable. Your breath is your best guide. Listen for a smooth, even flow. When counting the breath is required, gradually build up to your comfortable maximum count, not pushing to keep up with the count on the CD. **If your breath becomes restricted or choppy, it's usually an indication that you're pushing beyond your limits or holding a posture too long. Adjust your body to match your breath and <u>always</u> work within a comfortable range.**

Be aware that focusing on one part of the body can create tension in another. Working the lower back may in fact create an underlying level of tension in the neck and shoulders. Please use a blanket under your neck while lying on your back *(except in the **Bridge Pose**)*, particularly if you know you have a tendency to tighten in your upper body. You may also wish to try some of the neck and shoulder pose adaptations offered in the booklet.

> As you work your way through this program, be sure to listen to your body, listen to your breath, and pace yourself. Yoga is an invitation to step out of the habitual way you relate to yourself. It's an opportunity to treat yourself with compassion and care.

Create a dedicated space for your practice *(it doesn't have to be fancy, just a corner or room you can call your own for a period of time each day)*. This expresses your intention to take your healing seriously. Lighting candles or incense for ambiance, if that suits you, provides a nice addition but is not required. Make a clear and concise statement to yourself about your intention to heal. This will strengthen the potency of the practice and support your healing on an even deeper level. Statements that reinforce the potential for a pain-free back are the most effective *(ie: I experience my back as healed and whole or I choose to free myself of pain)*. You may also enjoy the suggested reflections that are at the end of each practice. Let these reflections inspire you and pique your curiosity to look more deeply into the intimate relationship between your body, mind, and heart.

May you find **The Essential Low Back Program** beneficial, and experience the optimum lower back health that so many others have enjoyed through yoga.

definition:
the Divine in me recognizes
and acknowledges the
Divine in you

namaste

THE ESSENTIAL LOW BACK PROGRAM
KEY IDEAS FOR PRACTICE:

- The CDs and accompanying booklet are *not intended to replace a medical evaluation* of your particular back condition. If you are experiencing lower back pain, please consult with a doctor before beginning this program.

- These practices are designed to build on one another. Although they do become increasingly more challenging, there is no need to hurry through them. Please listen to your body and progress at your own rate, supporting your body gently through its healing process.

- Always refer back to Practice Session 1, as your *"home base"* practice if you experience a flare up or feel particularly stressed or fatigued.

- Pain is usually the indicator we use for "something going wrong". Rather than seeing pain as a negative, think of it metaphorically as the body's way of getting your attention, like the smoke detector in your home. It's there to alert you of a problem and to call you to take action.

- *Relax.* Relaxation is the most crucial healing tool for managing pain, developing better flexibility, muscle tone, and increasing circulation.

- Yoga works from the inside out by slowing movement down, deepening the breath, and consciously using the breath to link movement with awareness.

- How you breathe literally dictates how you feel. Each of the practices in **The Essential Low Back Program** begins and ends with deep yoga breathing and all the movements are coordinated with the breath. The emphasis on the breath is intentional to teach you a very powerful tool for calming your own nervous system and unwinding yourself out of pain.

- If your breath becomes restricted of choppy, it's usually an indication that you're pushing beyond your limits or holding a posture too long. Adjust your body to match your breath and <u>always</u> work within a comfortable range.

- There isn't one supreme posture that will "fix" your back. What makes the difference is the relationship between the postures and how they are used to transform the neuro-muscular patterns of your movements.

- Extrapolating bits and pieces from one practice to another or performing the poses out of order puts you at risk of injury.

- As you work your way through this program, be sure to listen to your body, listen to your breath and pace yourself. Yoga is an invitation to step out of the habitual way you relate to yourself. It's an opportunity to treat yourself with compassion and care.

- Learning to activate the "pause button" creates *healing opportunities* that allow you to do things differently than you've done them in the past. The more healing opportunities you create, the healthier and more vibrant you'll feel.

- Healing happens when the body, mind and heart are aligned.

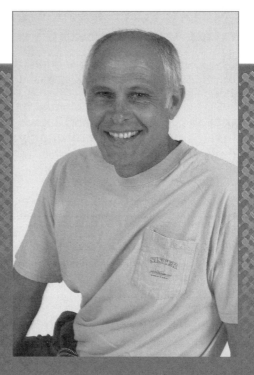

ARLEN

Two years ago, I was diagnosed with degenerative disc disease, stenosis, and scoliosis, all in the lumbar region. The result was severe sciatic pain in my right leg. I was advised to have surgery. At 55, I wasn't ready for a triple fusion, so I looked into some alternatives. After working with Viniyoga therapy for only a month, I now have more strength and flexibility than I've had in years. The yoga has 'awakened' some muscles I didn't know I had. My sciatic pain has been greatly reduced and I'm back on the golf course again.

PRACTICE SESSION 1

What you'll need for this practice:
A quiet space to practice, 45 minutes of uninterrupted
time, a couple of firm blankets, and a chair or bolster.

Introductory Breathing

Spread out one of the blankets and make yourself comfortable lying on the floor. Use the second blanket to give support to your neck if needed. Place the bolster or chair under your knees so your low back is in a neutral, relaxed position. Bring your attention to your breath, focusing first on your exhalation, drawing your belly in towards your spine from the bottom up, engaging your muscles from your lower abdominals to your upper abdominals as if squeezing toothpaste from the bottom of the tube. As you engage your abdomen this way, feel your lower back pressing gently into the floor. As you inhale, expand your chest and then your belly, filling your lungs from the top down. Allow your body to relax completely as you progressively deepen your breath for 10-12 breath cycles.

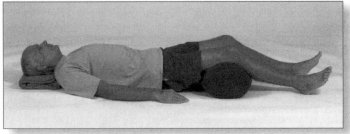

Introductory Breathing

Knee to Chest Pose – *One-Legged Variation*

Remove the bolster and place both feet on the floor, knees bent. As you exhale, fold your right knee into your chest and place your hand on your knee. As you inhale, expand your belly, keep your hands on your knee, and relax your knee away from your chest until your arm is straight. Keep your neck, shoulders, jaw, and throat relaxed. As you exhale, engage your abdominals and fold your knee once again into your chest. Repeat 4 times, then rest your right foot to the floor. Pause and feel the effect of the posture. Repeat the entire cycle with your left leg.

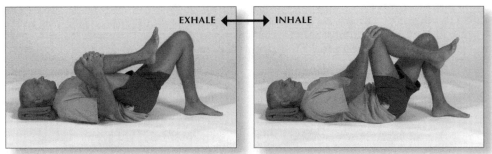

Knee to Chest Pose

Butterfly Pose – *2-Part Exhalation Variation*

Turn the soles of your feet to meet one another, allowing your hips to open. Inhale and expand your breath from your chest to belly. As you exhale, slowly squeeze your thighs together, engaging your belly and the muscles of your upper legs, pressing your lower back into the floor. Inhale and open your legs. Exhale slowly and consciously, stabilizing your pelvic girdle. Repeat this movement 6 times. Next, divide the exhalation movement and breath into two equal parts, like this: First, close your thighs halfway and exhale half the breath. Pause. Then continue to breathe out and bring your thighs together. Repeat for another 6 breath cycles keeping the exhalation movement slow and conscious and keeping all your pelvic muscles engaged.

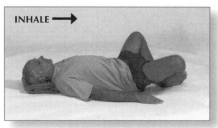

(a) Butterfly Pose

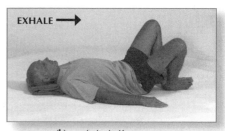

(b) • *exhale, half way pause*

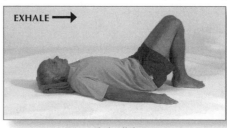

(c) • *exhale all the way*

*Wheel Pose – *2-Part Movement Variation*

Come onto your hands and knees and place a blanket under your knees for padding. Position your hands shoulder-width apart, directly below your shoulders, and place your knees hip-distance apart, directly below your hips. As you inhale, lift your tailbone, head, and chest into a back bend or "smile" position. As you exhale, engage your belly and draw in, tucking your tailbone under, stretching your hips halfway towards your heels to create a domed or rounded back. Release your chest and forehead to the floor. Pause. Inhale and lift forward. Repeat this cycle 3 times. For the next 3 cycles, stretch your hips all the way back so they rest on your heels. Forehead and forearms rest down as you release all the way back into **Child's Pose.**

Stay and rest in **Child's Pose** with your hips resting on your heels, arms either resting by your ears or by your heels and your forehead relaxed on the floor or blanket.

If you have a knee condition that prohibits you from kneeling, please do the seated, chair variation. For a full description of Seated Wheel or Seated Child's Pose, see pg. 64.

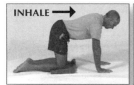

Wheel Pose

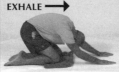

• *exhale, half way pause*

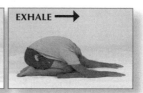

Resting Wheel/Child's Pose

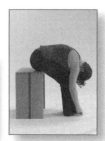

Seated Child's Pose
pg. 64

Cobra Pose

Come onto your belly with hands resting palms down just outside your shoulders, forearms on the floor, elbows by your ribs. Let your feet stretch back, tops of the feet on the floor. As you inhale, lift your chest without pushing with the hands, engaging your lower back and postural muscles so you can feel them gently tighten. Exhale and release your chest to the floor, turning your head to one side or resting your forehead down. Keep your neck relaxed as you work, tucking your chin slightly to avoid creating tension. Repeat a total of 6 times, progressively increasing the lift of your chest as your back will comfortably allow, without putting pressure on your hands.

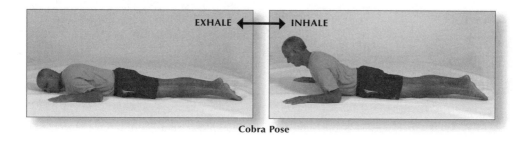

EXHALE ← → INHALE

Cobra Pose

Wheel Pose – *2-Part Movement Variation*

Come onto your hands and knees and place a blanket under your knees for padding. Position your hands shoulder-width apart, directly below your shoulders, and place your knees hip-distance apart, directly below your hips. As you inhale, lift your tailbone, head, and chest into a back bend or "smile" position. As you exhale, engage your belly and draw in, tucking your tailbone under, stretching your hips halfway towards your heels to create a domed or rounded back. Release your chest and forehead to the floor. Pause. Inhale and lift forward. Repeat this cycle 3 times. For the next 3 cycles, stretch your hips all the way back so they rest on your heels. Forehead and forearms rest down as you release all the way back into **Child's Pose**.

Stay and rest in **Child's Pose** with your hips resting on your heels, arms either resting by your ears or by your heels and your forehead relaxed on the floor or blanket.

> If you have a knee condition that prohibits you from kneeling, please do the seated, chair variation. For a full description of Seated Wheel, see pg. 64.

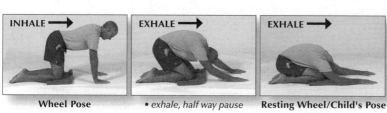

INHALE →   EXHALE →   EXHALE →

Wheel Pose   • *exhale, half way pause*   **Resting Wheel/Child's Pose**

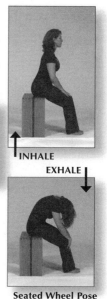

INHALE
EXHALE

Seated Wheel Pose
pg. 64

*The english names for postures may or may not correlate with the traditional Sanskrit names. They have been selected for simplicity and ease to accommodate those new to yoga. In particular, the pose called, **"The Wheel"** in The Essential Low Back Program, is traditionally translated as **"Ruddy-Goose Pose"**. In many yoga traditions, **"The Wheel"** refers to an intermediate to advanced back bend.*

Bridge Pose

Lie on your back with your knees bent and your feet hip-width apart, about 6-8 inches from your sit bones. Arms are relaxed by your side, and your head rests on the floor *without any support*. Inhale, press firmly down into your feet, lift your hips, and stretch into the front of your body. As you exhale, draw your belly in and curl your spine down, one vertebra at a time. Repeat 6 times.

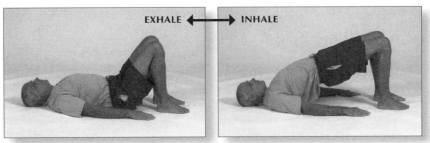

EXHALE ← → INHALE

Bridge Pose

Bridge Pose – *Alternate Arm Variation/Neck and Shoulder Release*

Inhale as you lift up into the **Bridge Pose**, raise your right arm and stretch it overhead to the floor behind you. As you exhale, bring your right arm down while turning your head to the left and curling your spine down to the resting position. As you inhale the next time, raise your left arm, turn head to center, and lift up. Exhale and bring your left arm down while turning your head to the right and curling your spine down to the resting position. Continue to alternate in this way until you've completed 3 cycles on each side.

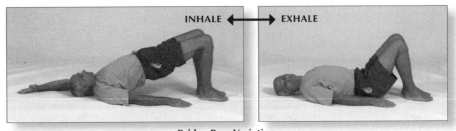

INHALE ← → EXHALE

Bridge Pose Variation

Knee to Chest Pose – *Two Legs*

Lie on your back and draw both knees up until you can place one hand on each knee. Exhale, folding your knees into your chest, stretching your lower back. As you inhale, release your knees back until they are an arm's length away from you *(feet stay off the floor)*. Repeat 3 times. Exhale, and divide the breath into two equal parts. Bring your knees in halfway as you release half the breath. Pause. Then continue to draw your knees in and press out the rest of your breath. Repeat this 2-part variation 3 times.

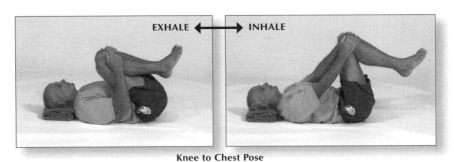

EXHALE ← → INHALE

Knee to Chest Pose

Relaxation

Lie down comfortably as you did in the beginning resting position. Place the bolster or chair under your knees, so your lower back can relax in a neutral position. Evenly spread your body across the floor. Let the whole body rest. Relax the breath, keeping the mind focused on the movement of the breath and the gentle release of muscular tension. Remain in this position for 3-5 minutes.

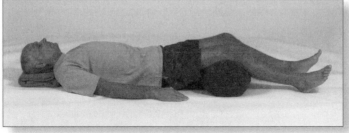

Relaxation and Lying Pranayama

Lying Pranayama/Deep Yoga Breathing

Begin to bring consciousness to the flow of the breath, making your breath more dynamic. As you breathe out, draw your belly in towards your spine from the bottom up, engaging the muscles from the lower abdominals to the upper abdominals, as if squeezing toothpaste from the bottom of the tube. As you engage your abdomen this way, feel your lower back pressing gently towards the floor. As you inhale, expand your chest and then your belly, filling your lungs from the top down. Deepen your breath progressively, staying focused on the extended exhale. Begin to divide your exhalation breath into 2 parts. Release half the breath as you draw your navel to your pubic bone. Pause. Then continue to engage your upper abdomen *(from navel to solar plexus)* as you press the second half of the breath out. Inhale freely, expanding from your chest to your belly. Repeat this 2-part exhalation for 8 breath cycles. Then, relax your breath and rest quietly for a few more minutes.

To come out, bring your knees into your chest, roll over onto your side, and press yourself up to a seated position. Sit quietly and observe the effect of your practice.

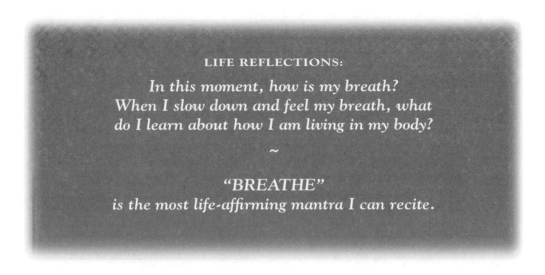

LIFE REFLECTIONS:

In this moment, how is my breath?
When I slow down and feel my breath, what
do I learn about how I am living in my body?

~

"BREATHE"
is the most life-affirming mantra I can recite.

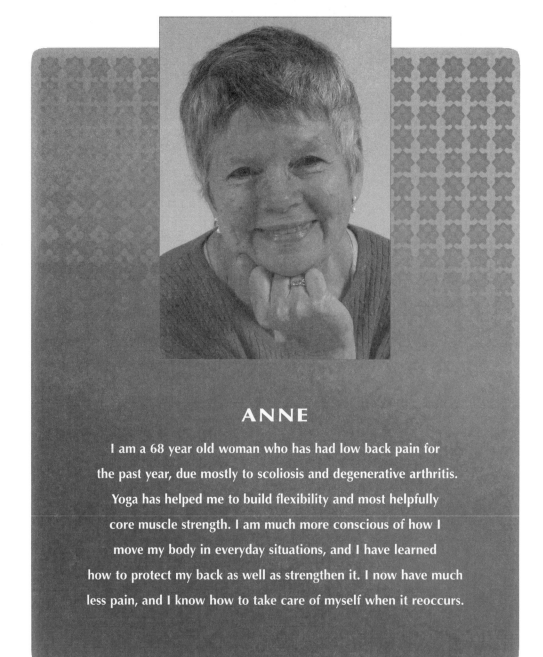

ANNE

I am a 68 year old woman who has had low back pain for
the past year, due mostly to scoliosis and degenerative arthritis.
Yoga has helped me to build flexibility and most helpfully
core muscle strength. I am much more conscious of how I
move my body in everyday situations, and I have learned
how to protect my back as well as strengthen it. I now have much
less pain, and I know how to take care of myself when it reoccurs.

PRACTICE SESSION 2

What you'll need for this practice:
A quiet space to practice, 60 minutes of uninterrupted time,
a yoga mat, a couple of firm blankets, and a chair or bolster.

*You may choose to do the Introductory Breathing lying down as in
Practice Session #1 or sitting in a chair in the Seated Mountain Pose*

Seated Mountain Pose

Place your sit bones at the edge of the seat, with your hips slightly elevated above
the height of your knees, feet planted firmly on the floor, and heels directly in line
with your knees. Align your shoulders above your hips, drop your chin slightly, and
rest your hands on your thighs. Begin to bring consciousness to the flow of your
breath, making your breath more dynamic. As you breathe out, draw your belly in
towards your spine from the bottom up, engaging your muscles from the lower
abdominals to your upper abdominals. As you engage your abdomen this way, feel
the arch of your lower back gently flatten, releasing tension. As you inhale, expand
your chest and then your belly, filling your lungs from the top down. Deepen your
breath progressively for 10-12 breath cycles.

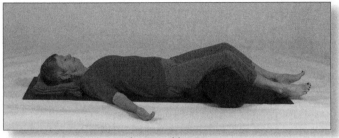

Lying Breathing Pose

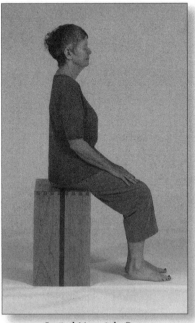

Seated Mountain Pose

Thunderbolt Pose – *Kneeling Forward Bend*

Stand on your knees with a folded blanket placed under your knees for cushioning. As you inhale, raise both arms in front of you and then over your head while continually lengthening your spine. As you exhale, sweep your arms out to the sides and down as you draw your abdominals in and bring your hips back to rest on your heels. Place the back of your hands onto your lower back and bring your head to the floor, releasing your neck as you fold forward to avoid tension. As you inhale, lift your spine, standing on your knees and reach out through your arms. Repeat the entire movement 6 times. *If you are unable to rest your head to the floor, you can use the bolster or chair for support. (option 2)*

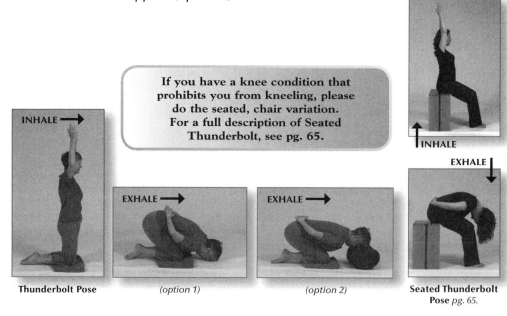

> If you have a knee condition that prohibits you from kneeling, please do the seated, chair variation. For a full description of Seated Thunderbolt, see pg. 65.

Thunderbolt Pose   (option 1)   (option 2)   Seated Thunderbolt Pose *pg. 65.*

Cobra – *Alternate Leg Variation*

Lie on your belly with hands resting just outside your shoulders, forearms on the floor, elbows by your ribs. Let your feet stretch back, tops of the feet on the floor. Inhale and without pushing into your arms, lift your chest and your right leg, engaging your lower back muscles so you can feel them gently tighten. Hold for a moment, then exhale and release your chest and leg to the floor, turning your head to the left or resting your forehead down. With your next inhale, lift your left leg and your chest, hold, then release on exhale, turning your head to the right. Continue, lifting your legs *(one at a time)* with your chest on inhale and releasing down as you exhale. Keep your neck relaxed as you work, tucking your chin slightly to avoid creating tension. Repeat 4 times on each side, slightly increasing the lift of your chest and leg as your back will comfortably allow.

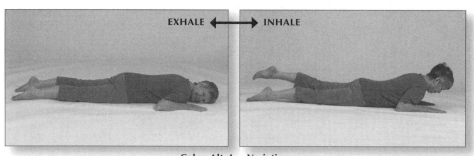

Cobra Alt. Leg Variation

Wheel Pose – *Progressive Exhale*

Come onto your hands and knees and place a blanket under your knees for support. Position your hands shoulder-width apart, directly below your shoulders, and place your knees hip-distance apart, directly below your hips. With your inhalation, lift your tailbone, head, and chest. As you exhale, engage your belly and stretch your hips back to your heels, counting your exhale in one second intervals for 4 counts. Repeat. Lengthen your exhale to 6 counts and repeat the movement for 2 breath cycles. Then lengthen your exhale to 8 counts and repeat the movement again for two breath cycles. Rest in **Child's Pose**.

> If you have a knee condition that prohibits you from kneeling, please do the seated, chair variation. For a full description of Seated Wheel, see pg. 64.

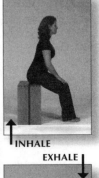

INHALE

EXHALE

Seated Wheel Pose
pg.64.

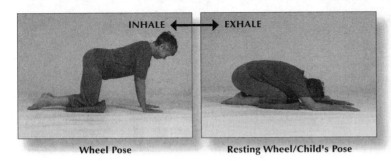

INHALE ←→ EXHALE

Wheel Pose

Resting Wheel/Child's Pose

Standing Mountain Pose

Stand on a mat that is cleared of props. Align your feet with one another, hip width apart. Lift your inner arches and balance the weight across the ball of your foot. Align your hips over your heels, bringing the weight back, and bring your shoulders directly in line over your hips. Draw your chin in slightly so your head moves back into alignment with your shoulders. Engage your belly to support your lower back and engage the postural muscles between your shoulders to support your upper body, neck, and head. Maintain a soft gaze as you focus your attention on your breath. Feel your chest expand and your spine lengthen with each inhalation. Use your Inner Core for support as you exhale and release tension from your body and mind. Stay for 10-12 breaths, cultivating a sense of grounding and inner balance.

Standing Mtn. Pose

Warrior Pose

Place your feet hip-width apart and step your right foot forward. Square your hips to the front of the room and turn your back foot slightly inward. Make sure your back heel is solidly grounded. As you inhale, bend your front knee into a standing lunge and sweep your arms out to the sides, keeping your shoulders relaxed and slightly in front of your hips. As you exhale, straighten your front leg and bring your arms back down by your side. Repeat this movement 3 times, then do the Lat-bar pull variation below.

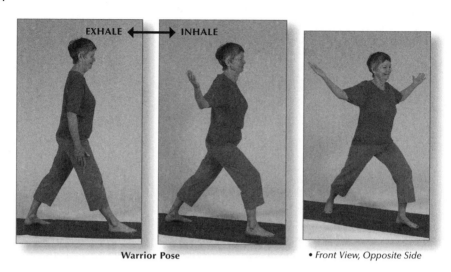

Warrior Pose • Front View, Opposite Side

Warrior Pose – *Lat-Bar Pull Variation*

As you inhale, bend your front knee into the lunge position and reach your arms forward and up, extending your spine. As you exhale, maintain the lunge position and bend your elbows, engaging your upper back postural muscles, pressing your chest forward. As you take this strong position in your upper body, engage your abdominals to stabilize and support your lower back. Keep your shoulders slightly forward of your hips, at a diagonal to avoid over-arching your lower back. Repeat the lat-bar pull movement in your arms 3 times, maintaining the lunge position in your legs. As you inhale, straighten your front leg and extend your arms forward and up. As you exhale, press your arms down and bring your feet together. Pause in **Mountain Pose** and then repeat the **Warrior** sequence on your other side. Return to **Mountain Pose**. Pause and feel the effect of the posture.

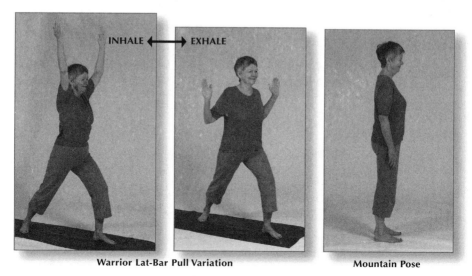

Warrior Lat-Bar Pull Variation   Mountain Pose

Chair Pose

Begin in **Standing Mountain Pose**. As you exhale, come into a half-squat, bending your knees. Bring your thighs parallel to the floor and fold forward, rotating in your hips, bringing your chest to your thighs. Your arms are relaxed toward the floor. Pause. As you inhale, press into your legs, and then leading with your chest, roll your shoulders back and come up fully into **Standing Mountain Pose**. Your arms remain relaxed, hands sliding up the legs. Repeat the movement with progressively longer exhalations: use a 4-count exhale for 2 repetitions, a 6-count exhale for 2 repetitions, and an 8-count exhale for 2 repetitions. When finished, stand in **Mountain Pose** for a few breaths and feel the effect of the posture.

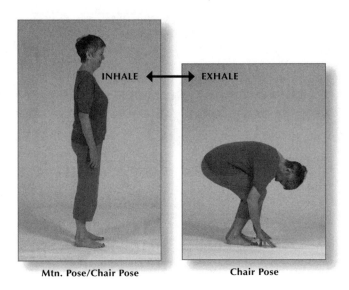

Mtn. Pose/Chair Pose   Chair Pose

Cobra Pose – *Widening Leg Variation*

Lie on your belly with hands resting palms down just outside your shoulders, forearms on the floor, elbows by your ribs. Begin with your feet hip-width apart. Let your feet stretch back, tops of the feet on the floor. Inhale and lift your chest maintaining a sense of length in the spine. Pause. Exhale and release your chest to the floor. Repeat this 2 times. Then widen the spread of your legs about 6 inches and repeat the same cobra lift 2 times. Progressively widen your legs twice more, 6 inches at a time, lifting up into **Cobra** 2 times in each position.

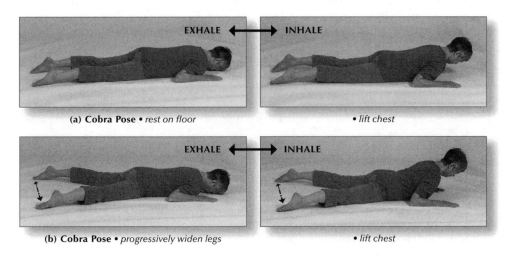

(a) **Cobra Pose** • *rest on floor*   • *lift chest*

(b) **Cobra Pose** • *progressively widen legs*   • *lift chest*

Wheel Pose – *Progressive Exhale*

Come onto your hands and knees and place a blanket under your knees for support. Position your hands shoulder-width apart, directly below your shoulders, and place your knees hip-distance apart, directly below your hips. With your inhalation, lift your tailbone, head, and chest. As you exhale, engage your belly and stretch your hips back to your heels, counting your exhale in one second intervals for 4 counts. Repeat. Lengthen your exhale to 6 counts and repeat the movement for 2 breath cycles. Then lengthen your exhale to 8 counts and repeat the movement again for two breath cycles. Rest in **Child's Pose**.

> If you have a knee condition that prohibits you from kneeling, please do the seated, chair variation. For a full description of Seated Wheel, see pg. 64.

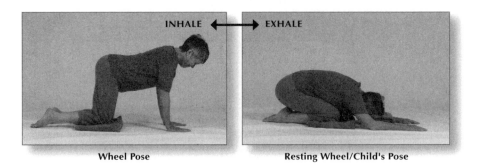

INHALE ←→ EXHALE

Wheel Pose   Resting Wheel/Child's Pose

Extended Leg Pose

Come onto your back, supporting your neck if needed. Bend your knees and place your feet on the floor. Settle into your breath, release any excess tension. Bring your right knee into your chest and place your hands just below the back of your right knee. With your inhalation, extend your right heel up towards the ceiling, straightening your right leg as much as you are able. As you exhale, bend your knee and draw your thigh into your chest. Repeat 4 times. Then hold your leg in the extended position and slowly circle your ankle 4-6 times in each direction. Keep your breath flowing naturally as you rotate your ankle. When you're finished, fold your knee into your chest as you exhale and then bring your foot to the floor. Pause and feel the effect of the posture. Repeat the sequence with your left leg.

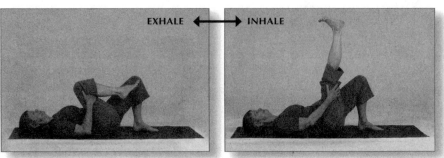

EXHALE ←→ INHALE

Extended Leg Pose

Bridge Pose – *Progressive Exhale*

Lie on your back with your knees bent and your feet hip-width apart, about 6-8 inches from your sit bones. Arms are relaxed by your side, and your head rests on the floor without any support. Inhale, press firmly down into your feet, lift your hips, and stretch into the front of your body. As you exhale, count to 4, drawing your belly in and curling your spine down one vertebra at a time. Repeat. Exhale out to 6 counts and repeat the movement for 2 breath cycles. Then lengthen your exhalation to 8 counts and repeat the movement again for two breath cycles. Rest and feel the effects of the posture.

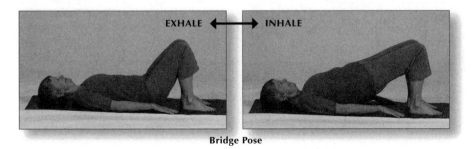

EXHALE ← → INHALE

Bridge Pose

Bridge Pose – *Alternate Arm Variation/Neck Shoulder Release*

Inhale, as you lift up into the **Bridge Pose**, raise your right arm and stretch it over-head to the floor behind you. As you exhale, bring your right arm down while turning your head to the left and curling your spine down to the resting position. As you inhale the next time, raise your left arm, turn head to center, and lift up. Exhale and bring your left arm down, turning your head to the right and curling your spine down to the resting position. Continue to alternate in this way until you've completed 3 times on each side.

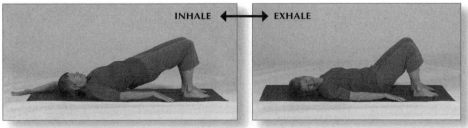

INHALE ← → EXHALE

Bridge Pose Variation

Knee to Chest Pose

Lie on your back and draw both knees up until you can place one hand on each knee. As you exhale, fold your knees into your chest, stretching your lower back. As you inhale, release your knees back until they are arms length away from you *(feet stay off the floor)*. Repeat 6 times, slowing the exhaled breath and movement.

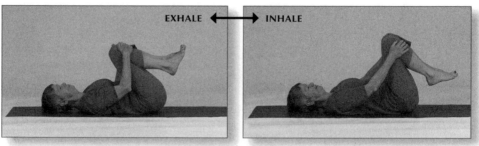

Knee to Chest Pose

Relaxation Pose

Arrange yourself comfortably and consciously on the floor. Place the bolster or chair under your knees so your low back can relax in a neutral position. Evenly spread your body across the floor, so you feel balanced right to left. Allow your whole body to rest. Relax your breath, keeping your mind focused on the movement of the breath and the gentle release of muscular tension. Remain in this position for 3-5 minutes.

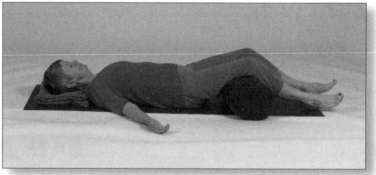

Relaxation Pose

Seated Pranayama/Deep Yoga Breathing

*(If you prefer to lie down for the breathing practice, you may stay in the **Relaxation Pose** to do the **Pranayama**.)*

Come into a **Seated Mountain Pose**, on a chair. Sit comfortably using a blanket as needed under your sitbones, so that you are able to hold your spine erect without great effort. Keeping your focus on your breath, expand your chest as you inhale. As you exhale, draw your belly in from your pubic bone to your navel, then continue to draw in from your navel to your solar plexus, flattening your lumbar curve as you press the breath out of your body.

Progressively lengthen your exhalation to 8 counts. Take several breath cycles to achieve this, keeping the breath long and smooth and the inhalation free and open. Once you've exhaled to the count of 8, divide the breath into two parts: For the first part, breathe out for 4 counts, drawing in from your lower abdominals *(pubic bone to navel)*. Pause. For the second part, breathe out for 4 counts, engaging your upper abdominals *(navel to solar plexus)*. Inhale and relax your belly as you expand from the top down. Repeat this 2-part exhale for 12 breath cycles. When you've completed your breathing practice, relax and breathe naturally. Stay for another 6–12 breaths, experiencing the effects of your practice.

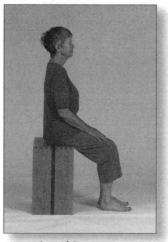

Seated Pranayama

LIFE REFLECTIONS:

When sensations of pain arise in me, how do I respond?
When feelings of peace and contentment arise in me,
how do I respond? Which do I attend to more?

~

As I look at the day or the week ahead,
have I left time to pause, time for stillness,
*time to breathe, time to **not**-do?*

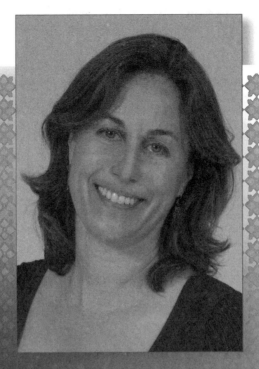

SHARON

For many years, I have experienced recurrent low back problems
that are disruptive to my life. I find that yoga is particularly helpful in
relieving my symptoms and has a longer-term positive effect.
Practicing yoga as I do now, with more awareness of how to activate my
inner core, as well as how to breathe and stretch properly,
has really helped to release my low back and de-stress my life.
A dedicated practice keeps my body balanced and pain-free and
is an important part in maintaining my health.

PRACTICE SESSION 3

What you'll need for this practice:
A quiet space to practice, 60 minutes of uninterrupted time,
a yoga mat, a couple of firm blankets, a chair or bolster,
and a yoga belt or a bathrobe sash.

Seated Mountain Pose

Place your sit bones at the edge of the seat, with your hips slightly elevated above the height of your knees, feet planted firmly on the floor, and heels directly in line with your knees. Align your shoulders above your hips, drop your chin slightly, and rest your hands on your thighs. Begin to bring consciousness to the flow of your breath, making your breath more dynamic. As you breathe out, draw your belly in towards your spine from the bottom up, engaging your muscles from your lower abdominals to your upper abdominals. As you engage your abdomen this way, feel the arch of your lower back gently flatten, releasing tension. As you inhale, expand your chest and then your belly, filling your lungs from the top down. Deepen your breath progressively for 10-12 breath cycles.

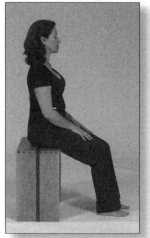
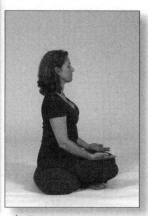

Seated Mountain Pose

Thunderbolt Pose — *Kneeling Forward Bend*

Stand on your knees with a folded blanket placed under your knees for cushioning. As you inhale, raise both arms in front of you and then over your head while continually lengthening your spine. As you exhale, sweep your arms out to the sides and down as you draw your abdominals in and bring your hips back to rest towards your heels.

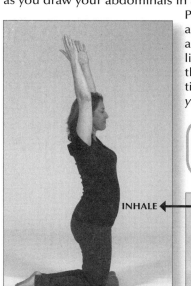

Place the back of your hands onto your lower back and bring your head to the floor, releasing your neck as you fold forward to avoid tension. As you inhale, lift your spine, standing on your knees and reach out through your arms. Repeat the entire movement 6 times. *If you are unable to rest your head to the floor, you can use your bolster or chair for support.*

> **If you have a knee condition that prohibits you from kneeling, please do the seated, chair variation. For a description of Seated Thunderbolt, see pg. 65.**

INHALE ◄――――► EXHALE

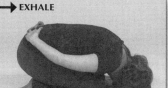
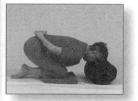

Thunderbolt Pose • *use a bolster to support your head if necessary*

Cobra – *Alternate Leg Variation*

Lie on your belly with hands resting just outside your shoulders, forearms on the floor, elbows by your ribs. Let your feet stretch back, tops of your feet on the floor. Inhale and without pushing into your arms, lift your chest and your right leg, engaging your lower back muscles so you can feel them gently tighten. Hold for a moment, then exhale and release your chest and leg to the floor, turning your head to the left or resting your forehead down. With your next inhale, lift your left leg and your chest, hold, then release on exhale, turning your head to the right. Continue, lifting your legs *(one at a time)* with your chest on inhale and releasing down as you exhale. Keep your neck relaxed as you work, tucking your chin slightly to avoid creating tension. Repeat 4 times on each side, slightly increasing the lift of your chest and leg as your back will comfortably allow.

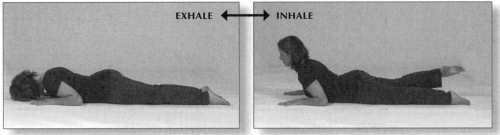

EXHALE ← → INHALE

Cobra Alt. Leg Variation

Wheel – *Hold After Exhale*

Come onto your hands and knees and place a blanket under your knees for padding. Position your hands shoulder-width apart, directly below your shoulders, and place your knees hip-distance apart, directly below your hips. As you inhale, lift your tailbone, head, and chest. As you exhale, engage your belly, draw in, tuck your tailbone under, and stretch your hips towards your heels, releasing your chest and forehead to the floor. Pause for 2-3 seconds in the stillness. Then inhale and lift forward. Repeat 6 times, exploring the stillness after the exhaled breath and allowing your whole body to release and relax more fully with each consecutive cycle.

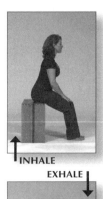

INHALE

EXHALE

> If you have a knee condition that prohibits you from kneeling, please do the seated, chair variation. For a full description of Seated Wheel, see pg 64.

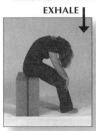

Seated Wheel Pose
pg 64

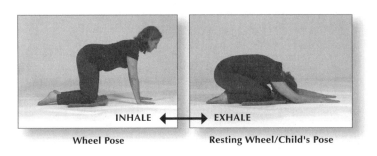

INHALE ← → EXHALE

Wheel Pose   Resting Wheel/Child's Pose

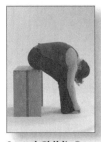

Seated Child's Pose

Standing Forward Bend

Stand on your mat in **Mountain Pose** and check your alignment. Inhale in this position to lengthen your spine. As you exhale, bend your knees slightly and fold forward, while maintaining a straight spine. Once you stretch down half-way towards the floor allow your back to round. Slide your hands down your legs for a comfortable stretch and let your head completely go. As you inhale, press into your legs and lift up as if coming out of **Chair Pose**—legs strong, shoulders rolled back, chest lifted. Repeat 4 times and then stay in the **Forward Bend** for 3-4 breaths to deepen the stretch on the back of your body. Come up as you inhale, engaging your back muscles and your abdominals to provide good postural support for your back. If your back feels strained with your hands resting on your legs, place your hands on the seat of the chair or on the bolster for support.

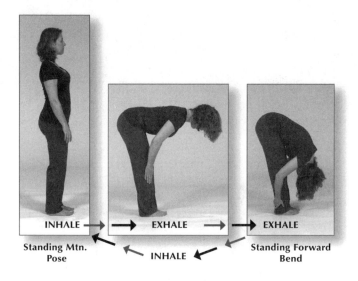

INHALE → EXHALE → EXHALE

Standing Mtn. Pose ← INHALE ← Standing Forward Bend

Asymmetrical Standing Forward Bend

Place your feet hip-width apart and step your right foot forward. Square your hips to the front of the room and turn your back foot slightly inward. Check that your back heel is solidly grounded. Inhale and create a **Mountain Pose** extension in your spine. As you exhale, fold forward over your front leg, rotating from your hips, not folding from your waist. Relax your head and neck. Keep your front knee bent just enough to accommodate tightness in the back of your leg. As you inhale, straighten your spine and lift up using your abdominal muscles, spinal muscles, and legs for support. Repeat 3 times, then stay in the pose for 3 breaths, deepening into the stretch. Inhale and come up, then return to **Mountain Pose**. Pause and feel the effect of the posture. Change sides and repeat the sequence.

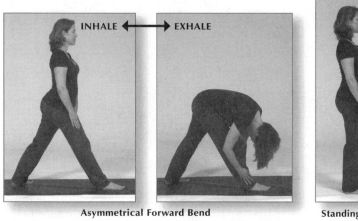

INHALE ← → EXHALE

Asymmetrical Forward Bend

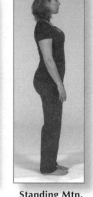

Standing Mtn. Pose

Cobra — *Swimmer's Variation*

Come onto your belly with hands resting just outside your shoulders, forearms on the floor, elbows by your ribs. Begin with your feet hip-width apart. Let your feet stretch back, tops of the feet on the floor. Inhale and lift your chest and your legs, straddling your legs wide apart. Pause. Exhale and squeeze your thighs together, keeping your chest and legs lifted. Release and relax your chest and legs to the floor. Take a breath in the resting position, then repeat the lift, straddle and squeeze movement for a total of 6 cycles. As you feel strong enough, try 2 or 3 repetitions of the straddle and squeeze movement in a row without resting. *Build strength gradually with this posture. Don't push.*

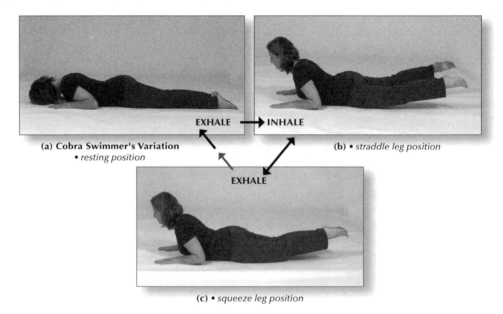

EXHALE → INHALE

(a) Cobra Swimmer's Variation
• *resting position*

(b) • *straddle leg position*

EXHALE

(c) • *squeeze leg position*

Wheel — *Hold After Exhale*

Come onto your hands and knees and place a blanket under your knees for padding. Position your hands shoulder-width apart, directly below your shoulders, and place your knees hip-distance apart, directly below your hips. As you inhale, lift your tailbone, head, and chest. As you exhale, engage your belly, draw in, tuck the tailbone under, and stretch your hips towards your heels, releasing your chest and forehead to the floor. Pause for 2-3 seconds in the stillness. Then inhale and lift forward. Repeat 6 times, exploring the stillness after the exhaled breath and allowing your whole body to release and relax more fully with each consecutive cycle.

> **If you have a knee condition that prohibits you from kneeling, please do the seated, chair variation. For a full description of Seated Wheel, see pg. 64.**

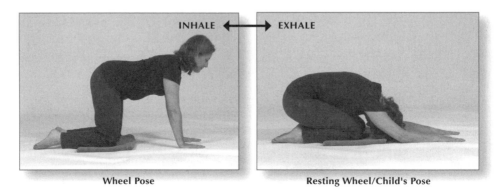

INHALE ← → EXHALE

Wheel Pose

Resting Wheel/Child's Pose

Extended Leg Pose – *With Belt*

(a) Lie on your back with your knees bent, feet on the floor. Exhale and bring your right knee into your chest and place the belt around the ball of your right foot. As you inhale, extend your right leg fully, maintaining a relaxed grip on the belt with your hands. As you exhale, bend your right knee towards your chest. Continue to work this way for 4-6 breaths.

(b) Next, keeping the belt looped around your foot, hold it with your right hand and stabilize your left hip *(ground firmly down through your left foot and hip)*. As you inhale, sweep your right leg out to the right, stretching your inner thigh. As you exhale, draw your right leg up to center and then to the left to stretch your outer hip and leg. To increase the stretch on your outer thigh, rotate your thigh inward slightly and bring your right heel towards your left shoulder.

Repeat this windshield-wiper action 4-6 times. Then bring your right leg to center, release the belt, and bring both knees into your chest for **Knee to Chest Pose** *(see below)*. Repeat on second side.

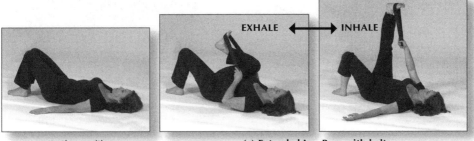

• *starting position*　　　　　**(a) Extended Leg Pose with belt**

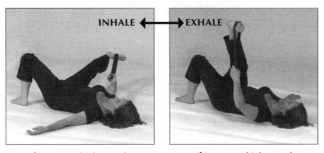

(b) • *inner thigh stretch*　　　　**(b)** • *outer thigh stretch*

Knee to Chest Pose

Lie on your back and draw both knees up until you can place one hand on each knee. As you exhale, fold your knees into your chest, stretching your lower back. As you inhale, release your knees back until they are arms length away from you *(feet stay off the floor)*. Repeat 6 times, slowing the exhaled breath and movement.

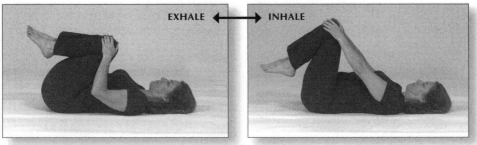

Knee to Chest Pose

Butterfly Pose – *2 Part Exhalation Variation*

Turn the soles of your feet to meet one another, allowing your hips to open. Inhale and expand your breath from your chest to your belly. As you exhale, slowly squeeze your thighs together, engaging your belly and the muscles of your upper leg, pressing your lower back into the floor. Inhale and open your legs. Exhale slowly and consciously, stabilizing your pelvic girdle. Repeat this movement 6 times. Next, divide the exhalation movement and breath into two equal parts, like this: First, close your thighs halfway and exhale half your breath. Pause. Then continue to breathe out and bring your thighs together. Repeat for another 6 breath cycles keeping the exhalation movement slow and conscious and keeping all your pelvic muscles engaged.

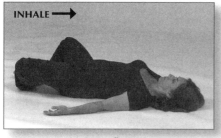

(a) **Butterfly Pose**

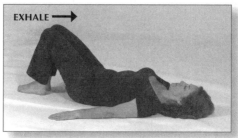

(b) • *exhale, half way pause*

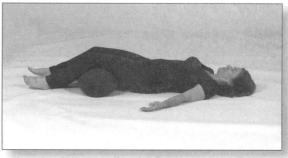

(c) • *exhale all the way*

Relaxation Pose

Arrange yourself comfortably and consciously on the floor. Place the bolster or chair under your knees so your low back can relax in a neutral position. Evenly spread your body across the floor, so you feel balanced right to left. Allow your whole body to rest. Relax your breath, keeping your mind focused on the movement of your breath and the gentle release of muscular tension. Remain in this position for 3-5 minutes.

Relaxation Pose

Seated Pranayama/Deep Yoga Breathing

*(If you prefer to lie down for the breathing practice, you may stay in the **Relaxation Pose** to do the **Pranayama**.)*

Come into a **Seated Mountain Pose**, either in a chair or in a simple cross-legged position on the floor. Sit comfortably using a blanket or bolster under your sitbones so that you are able to hold your spine erect without great effort. Keeping your focus on your breath, expand your chest as you inhale. As you exhale, draw your belly in from your pubic bone to your navel, then continue to draw in from your navel to your solar plexus, flattening your lumbar curve as you press the breath out of your body.

Progressively lengthen your exhalation to 8 counts. Take several breath cycles to achieve this, keeping the breath long and smooth and the inhalation free and open. Once you've exhaled to the count of 8, divide the breath into two parts: For the first part, breathe out for 4 counts, drawing in from your lower abdominals *(pubic bone to navel)*. Pause. For the second part, breathe out for 4 counts, engaging your upper abdominals *(navel to solar plexus)*. Inhale and relax your belly as you expand from the top down. Repeat this 2-part exhale for 12 breath cycles. When you've completed your breathing practice, relax and breathe naturally. Stay for another 6-12 breaths, experiencing the effects of your practice.

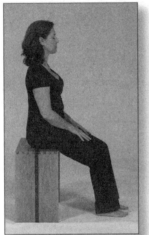
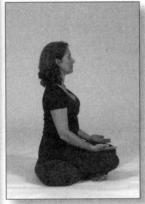

Seated Pranayama

LIFE REFLECTIONS:

How can I move through my day with a Mountain Pose awareness?

How does this awareness change how I perceive myself and the world around me?

~

When I feel disjointed and ungrounded, what are the tools I can use to bring me back into balance?

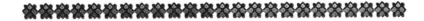

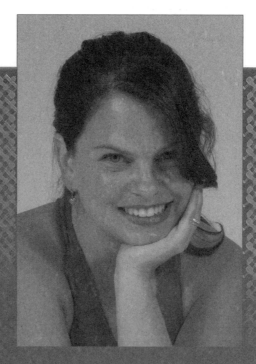

TARAN

After experiencing a car accident in my teens, my back
became a chronic issue. I tried many healing modalities but
experienced only temporary relief of my discomfort. It wasn't
until I discovered yoga that my back actually began to heal.
To my surprise, yoga not only helped stabilize my sacrum
and relieve my upper and lower back pain, but it also
brought balance and clarity into my life.
I now teach yoga and value the tools that allow
me and my students to continue to strengthen and
challenge our bodies, minds, and spirits.

PRACTICE SESSION 4

What you'll need for this practice:
A quiet space to practice, 60 minutes of uninterrupted time,
a yoga mat, a couple of firm blankets, and a chair or bolster.

Seated Mountain Pose

Place your sit bones at the edge of the seat, with your hips slightly elevated above the height of your knees, feet planted firmly on the floor, and heels directly in line with your knees. Align your shoulders above your hips, drop your chin slightly, and rest your hands on your thighs. Begin to bring consciousness to the flow of your breath, making your breath more dynamic. As you breathe out, draw your belly in towards your spine from the bottom up, engaging your muscles from your lower abdominals to your upper abdominals. As you engage your abdomen this way, feel the arch of your lower back gently flatten, releasing tension. As you inhale, expand your chest and then your belly, filling your lungs from the top down. Deepen your breath progressively for 10-12 breath cycles.

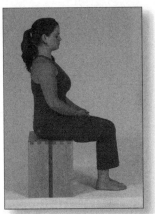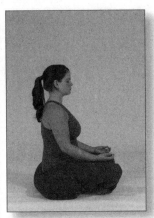

Seated Mountain Pose

Wheel Pose – *2 Part Movement Variation*

Come onto your hands and knees and place a blanket under your knees for padding. Position your hands shoulder-width apart, directly below your shoulders, and place your knees hip-distance apart, directly below your hips. As you inhale, lift your tailbone, head, and chest into a back bend or "smile" position. As you exhale, engage your belly and draw in, tucking your tailbone under, and stretching your hips halfway towards your heels to create a domed or rounded back. Release your chest and forehead to the floor. Pause. Inhale and lift forward. Repeat this cycle 3 times. For the next 3 cycles, stretch your hips all the way back so they rest on your heels. Forehead and forearms rest down as you release all the way back into **Child's Pose.**

Stay and rest in **Child's Pose** with heels resting to your hips, hands either resting by your ears or by your heels and your forehead relaxed on the floor or blanket.

> If you have a knee condition that prohibits you from kneeling, please do the seated, chair variation. For a full description of Seated Wheel, see pg. 64.

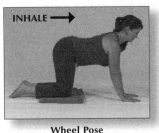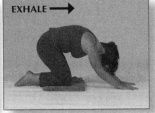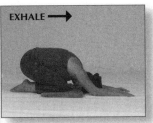

Wheel Pose **Resting Wheel/Child's Pose**

Cobra Pose — *Widening Leg Variation*

Lie on your belly with hands resting palms down just outside your shoulders, fore-arms on the floor, elbows by your ribs. Begin with your feet hip-width apart. Let your feet stretch back, tops of the feet on the floor. Inhale and lift your chest. Pause. Exhale and release your chest to the floor. Repeat this 2 times. Then widen the spread of your legs about 6 inches and repeat the same cobra lift 2 times. Progressively widen your legs twice more, 6 inches at a time, lifting up into **Cobra** 2 times in each position.

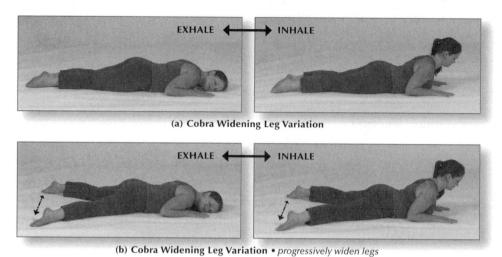

(a) **Cobra Widening Leg Variation**

(b) **Cobra Widening Leg Variation** • *progressively widen legs*

Cobra — *Swimmer's Variation*

Come onto your belly with hands resting just outside your shoulders, forearms on the floor, elbows by your ribs. Begin with your feet hip-width apart. Let your feet stretch back, tops of your feet on the floor. Inhale and lift your chest and your legs, straddling your legs wide apart. Pause. Exhale and squeeze your thighs together, keeping your chest and legs lifted. Release and relax your chest and legs to the floor. Take a breath in the resting position, then repeat the lift, straddle and squeeze movement for a total of 6 cycles. As you feel strong enough, try 2 or 3 repetitions of the straddle and squeeze movement in a row without resting. *Build strength gradually with this posture. Don't push.*

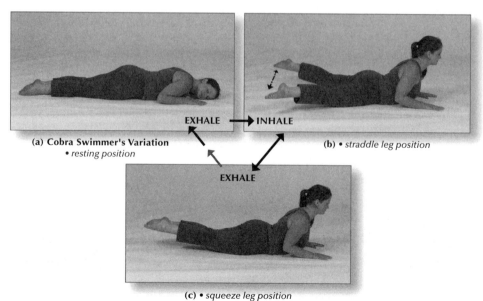

(a) **Cobra Swimmer's Variation**
• *resting position*

(b) • *straddle leg position*

(c) • *squeeze leg position*

Wheel Pose – *2-Part Movement variation*

Come onto your hands and knees and place a blanket under your knees for padding. Position your hands shoulder-width apart, directly below your shoulders, and place your knees hip-distance apart, directly below your hips. As you inhale, lift your tail-bone, head, and chest into a back bend or "smile" position. As you exhale, engage your belly and draw in, tucking your tailbone under, stretching your hips halfway towards your heels to create a domed or rounded back. Release your chest and forehead to the floor. Pause. Inhale and lift forward. Repeat this cycle 3 times. For the next 3 cycles, stretch your hips all the way back so they rest on your heels. Forehead and forearms rest down as you release all the way back into **Child's Pose.**

Stay and rest in **Child's Pose** with heels resting to your hips, arms either resting by your ears or by your heels and your forehead relaxed on the floor or blanket.

If you have a knee condition that prohibits you from kneeling, please do the seated, chair variation. For a full description of Seated Wheel, see pg. 64.

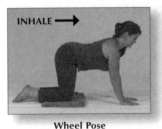
INHALE ➡

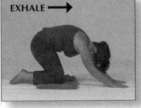
EXHALE ➡

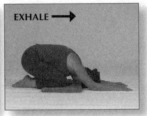
EXHALE ➡

Wheel Pose

Resting Wheel/Child's Pose

Kneeling Lunge

Kneel on a blanket with your hands on the floor and bring your right leg forward. Position your right leg so your shin is perpendicular to the floor. Move your left knee back until you feel a deep stretch on the front on your left thigh and hip. Lift your chest slightly, keeping light pressure on your hands. When you feel balanced, bring your hands up to rest on your right knee. Continue to drop into the stretch on your left hip and groin. Support your lower back by drawing your abdominals in. Keep your breath moving as you stay in the position for 3-4 breath cycles.

When you next inhale, lean slightly forward and reach up with your left arm to increase the stretch on your left side. As you exhale, press your left arm down. Repeat this arm movement 3 times, then stay and hold the stretch with your left arm up for 3 more breaths. Release out of the stretch and bring your right leg back. Kneel here. Pause and feel the effect of the pose.

If you're unable to kneel, work with the back leg lifted off the floor or in the chair variation of the lunge, as described on pg. 65.

Repeat the **Kneeling Lunge** sequence with your left leg forward and your right arm up.

Fold back and rest in **Child's Pose.**

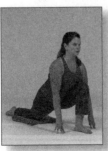

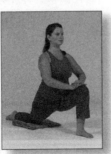

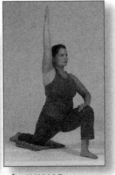

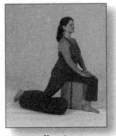

(a) Kneeling Lunge

(b) EXHALE ⬅➡ INHALE

Kneeling Lunge Chair Variation

Knees to Chest and Extended Leg Pose Variations

(a) Coming to lie on your back, take a few repetitions of **Knees to Chest Pose** with hands around your knees.

(b) Now, rest your arms by your side, and repeat the movement working from the abdominal core. Exhale, draw your knees into your chest. Hold there 2-3 seconds. Inhale and relax your knees back four to six inches *(feet off the floor, lower back flat to the floor)*. Repeat this movement 4-6 times. Keep your neck, jaw, and throat relaxed, shoulders soft.

(c) With your next inhalation, extend your legs, pressing your heels up towards the ceiling *(keep your palms pressing down by your side)*, exhale and fold your knees to your chest, holding for 2-3 seconds after you breathe out. Repeat this movement 3 times.

(d) Add the arms to this leg extension movement. Stretching your arms overhead and extending your legs on inhale, fold knees to chest and press your arms down by your side as you exhale, for another 3 repetitions. If this movement feels too challenging for your back, please work with variations b or c and build to your comfort. When you complete the repetitions, bring your feet to the floor. Pause and feel.

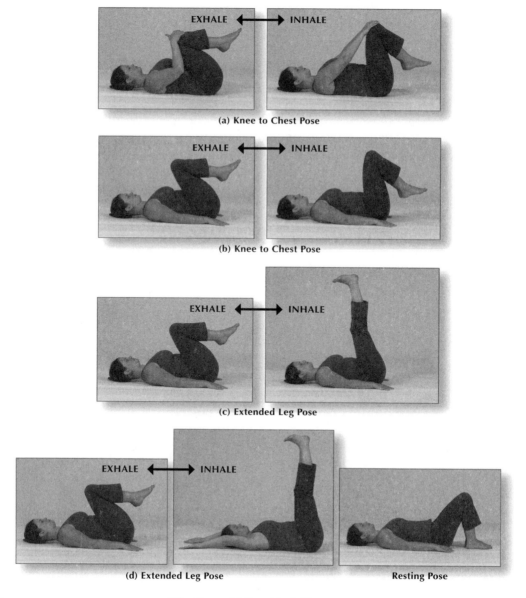

(a) Knee to Chest Pose

(b) Knee to Chest Pose

(c) Extended Leg Pose

(d) Extended Leg Pose   Resting Pose

Side-Lying Hip Strengtheners

(a) Lie on your right side with your knees bent. Place a folded blanket under your head and neck for support. Stack your hips so they are in line with each other and observe a **Mountain Pose** alignment from your crown to your tailbone. As you inhale, engage the muscles of your outer left thigh and hip and lift your left thigh off of your right. Hold for 2-3 seconds, then exhale and slowly lower your left leg down. Repeat 3 times.

(b) Now, keeping your right leg bent, straighten your left leg to the 6:00 position so that your left heel is in **Mtn. Pose** alignment with your spine and head.

Rotate your left thigh in *(knee and toes point down)*. Inhale and lift your leg, hold in position, then exhale and release down. Repeat 3 times.

Then, bring your leg forward about 6 inches *(5:00 position)* and repeat the leg lift movement coordinated with your breath. Continue this process in the 4:00 and 3:00 positions, 3 times each.

(c) Working with a circular movement in your hip, as if drawing a ½ circle with your whole leg, moving through positions 6:00-3:00, 3-4 times. Then reverse the direction. Circulate your breath as you rotate your leg. If you feel a lot of fatigue in the muscles of your hip and buttocks, work with baby circles, keeping your knee bent creating less load on your hip joint. Gradually straighten your leg as you build strength. After completing the series, come and rest on your back. Pause, before shifting onto your left side to work your right hip rotators. *When working with these, please build gradually, working the muscles to fatigue, not beyond. Rest as needed.*

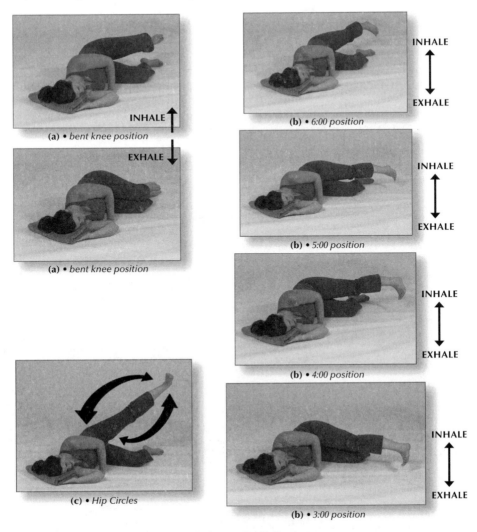

INHALE
EXHALE

INHALE

EXHALE

(a) • bent knee position

(b) • 6:00 position

(a) • bent knee position

INHALE

EXHALE

(b) • 5:00 position

INHALE

EXHALE

(b) • 4:00 position

INHALE

EXHALE

(c) • Hip Circles

(b) • 3:00 position

The Essential Low Back Program

Leg Cradle Stretch

Rest on your back with your knees bent. Cross your right ankle over your left knee. Bring your left foot off the floor and hold behind the back of your left thigh *(if comfortable for your neck and shoulders)* or hold your right shin and ankle with your hands. As you exhale, bring your right shin in towards your chest. As you inhale, rock your legs back until they are arm's length away. Repeat 3-4 times, then gently circle in your hips, to deepen the feeling of stretch in your hip rotators. Circle in one direction 3-4 breaths then rotate your hips in the other direction. Pause between sides, resting your feet on the floor. Then, cross your left ankle over your right knee, and take the **Leg Cradle** stretch on your other side.

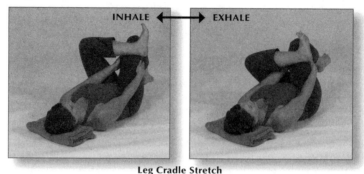

Leg Cradle Stretch

Knee to Chest Pose

Lie on your back and draw both knees up until you can place one hand on each knee. As you exhale, fold your knees into your chest, stretching your lower back. As you inhale, release your knees back until they are an arm's length away from you (feet stay off the floor). Repeat 3 times. Then divide the exhalation movement and breath into two equal parts. Bring your knees in halfway as you release half your breath. Pause. Then continue to draw your knees in and press out the rest of your breath. Repeat this 2-part variation 3 times.

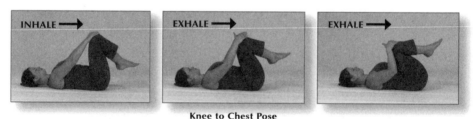

Knee to Chest Pose

Relaxation Pose

Arrange yourself comfortably and consciously on the floor. Place the bolster or chair under your knees so your low back can relax in a neutral position. Evenly spread your body across the floor, so you feel balanced right to left. Allow your whole body to rest. Relax your breath, keeping your mind focused on the movement of the breath and the gentle release of muscular tension. Remain in this position for 3-5 minutes.

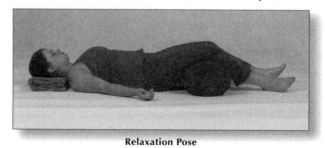

Relaxation Pose

Seated Pranayama/Deep Yoga Breathing

Come into a **Seated Mountain Pose**, either in a chair or in a simple cross-legged position on the floor. Sit comfortably using a blanket or bolster under your sitbones so that you are able to hold your spine erect without great effort. Keeping your focus on your breath, expand your chest as you inhale. As you exhale, draw your belly in from your pubic bone to your navel, then continue to draw in from your navel to your solar plexus, flattening your lumbar curve as you press the breath out of your body.

Progressively lengthen your exhalation to 8 counts. Take several breath cycles to achieve this, keeping the breath long and smooth and the inhalation free and open. Once you've exhaled to the count of 8, divide the breath into two parts: For the first part, breathe out for 4 counts, drawing in from your lower abdominals *(pubic bone to navel)*. Pause. For the second part, breathe out for 4 counts, engaging your upper abdominals *(navel to the solar plexus)*. Inhale and relax your belly as you expand from the top down. Repeat this 2-part exhale for 12 breath cycles. When you've completed your breathing practice, relax and breathe naturally. Stay for another 6-12 breaths, experiencing the effects of your practice.

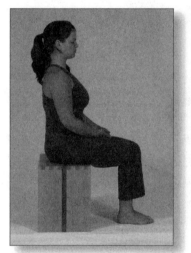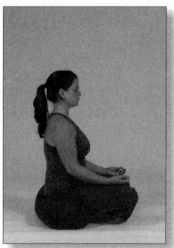

Seated Pranayama

LIFE REFLECTIONS:

*The future and the past are merely figments
of my imagination, the only time that exists is NOW*

How can I be radically present in this moment?

~

*What will it cost me if I stop?
What will it cost me if I don't?*

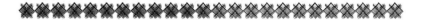

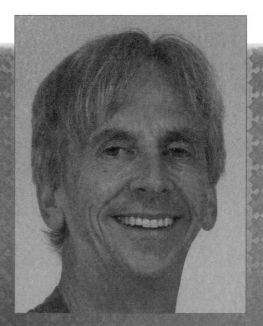

HARVEY

In the fall of 2003, while playfully racing my 13-year old daughter to the mall entry-way, I slipped on a wet tile and landed hard on my hip. At the time, I was amazed that I seemingly was not hurt. But a month later I had intense back and sciatic nerve pain. I couldn't walk more than a hundred yards before I was in tears. I couldn't sit for more than 15 minutes before it felt like 15 hours. OTC or prescribed pain killers did nothing except give me side effects. Physical therapy made it worse! I had to have surgery to move my ruptured disc off the severely inflamed nerve, but a month later I ruptured it again and had to repeat the surgery. My surgeon said that if I ruptured it a third time my vertebrae would have to be fused. And I was still miserable. At times I lost feeling in my leg and my knee would nearly collapse. Cortisone injections were painful and only temporarily effective. I thought I would have to quit my job. The pain was so bad that after a year and a half, I began to wonder how I was going to make the rest of my life worth living.

Finally, out of desperation, I listened to a co-worker who insisted that Viniyoga could help me. Until then, I thought that yoga was too far out from mainstream medicine, or just too 'New Age', to be effective. But, when I asked my surgeon about it he was enthusiastic and said he wished more of his patients would take up yoga as part of their recovery, as long as the practice was not too intense. In June of 2005, I signed up for an intro series and had a private evaluation to get me started on a home prac-tice. Viniyoga has taught me postural alignment and how to move safely. Regular home practice gradually relieved my back and sciatic nerve pain completely. Class participation has increased my flexibility and body-awareness to make re-injury much less likely. Study of yoga philosophy has helped me reduce stress and understand the importance of maintaining balance in all aspects of my life. I truly feel transformed.

> ## PRACTICE SESSION 5
> *What you'll need for this practice:*
> *A quiet space to practice, 60 minutes of uninterrupted time,*
> *a yoga mat, a couple of firm blankets, and a chair or bolster.*

Seated Mountain Pose

Place your sit bones at the edge of the seat, with your hips slightly elevated above the height of your knees, feet planted firmly on the floor, and heels directly in line with your knees. Align your shoulders above your hips, drop your chin slightly, and rest your hands on your thighs. Begin to bring consciousness to the flow of your breath, making your breath more dynamic. As you breathe out, draw your belly in towards your spine from the bottom up, engaging the muscles from your lower abdominals to your upper abdominals. As you engage your abdomen this way, feel the arch of your lower back gently flatten, releasing tension. As you inhale, expand your chest and then your belly, filling your lungs from the top down. Deepen your breath progressively for 10-12 breath cycles.

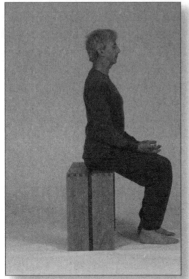
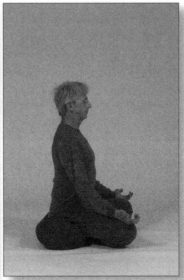

Seated Mountain Pose

Thunderbolt Pose

Stand on your knees with a folded blanket placed under your knees for cushioning. As you inhale, raise both arms in front of you and then over your head while continually lengthening your spine. As you exhale, sweep your arms out to the sides and down as you draw your abdominals in and bring your hips back to rest towards your heels. Place the back of your hands onto your lower back and bring your head to the floor, releasing your neck as you fold forward to avoid tension. As you inhale, lift your spine, standing on your knees and reach out through your arms. Repeat the entire movement 6 times. *If you are unable to rest your head to the floor, you can use your bolster or chair for support.*

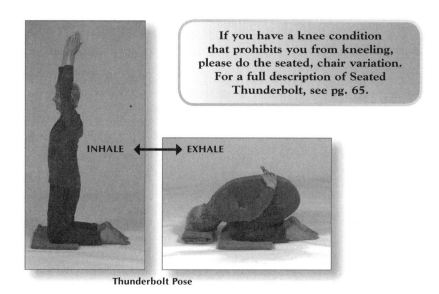

If you have a knee condition that prohibits you from kneeling, please do the seated, chair variation. For a full description of Seated Thunderbolt, see pg. 65.

INHALE ← → EXHALE

Thunderbolt Pose

Cobra – *Alternate Leg Variation*

Lie on your belly with hands resting just outside your shoulders, forearms on the floor, elbows by your ribs. Let your feet stretch back, tops of your feet on the floor. Inhale and without pushing into your arms, lift your chest and your right leg, engaging your lower back muscles so you can feel them gently tighten. Hold for a moment, then exhale and release your chest and leg to the floor, turning your head to the left or resting your forehead down. With your next inhale, lift your left leg and your chest, hold, then release on exhale, turning your head to the right. Continue, lifting your legs *(one at a time)* with your chest on inhale and releasing down as you exhale. Keep your neck relaxed as you work, tucking your chin slightly to avoid creating tension. Repeat 4 times on each side, slightly increasing the lift of your chest and leg as your back will comfortably allow.

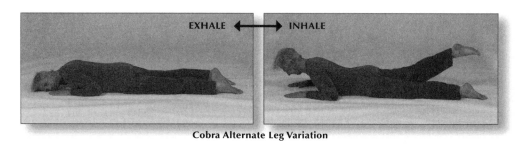

EXHALE ← → INHALE

Cobra Alternate Leg Variation

Wheel Pose – *Progressive Exhale*

Come onto your hands and knees and place a blanket under your knees for padding. Position your hands shoulder-width apart, directly below your shoulders, and place your knees hip-distance apart, directly below your hips. With your inhalation, lift your tailbone, head, and chest. As you exhale, engage your belly and stretch your hips back to your heels, counting your exhale in one second intervals for 4 counts. Repeat. Lengthen your exhalation to 6 counts and repeat the movement for 2 breath cycles. Then lengthen your exhalation to 8 counts and repeat the movement again for two breath cycles. Rest in **Child's Pose.**

> **If you have a knee condition that prohibits you from kneeling, please do the seated, chair variation. For a full description of Seated Wheel, see pg. 64.**

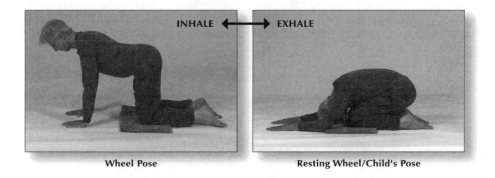

INHALE ⬅ ➡ EXHALE

Wheel Pose   Resting Wheel/Child's Pose

Standing Mountain Pose

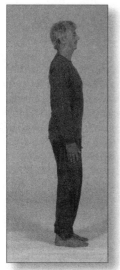

Standing
Mountain Pose

Stand on a mat that is cleared of props. Align your feet with one another, hip width apart. Lift your inner arches and balance the weight across the ball of your foot. Align your hips over your heels, bringing the weight back, and bring your shoulders directly in line over your hips. Draw your chin in slightly so your head moves back into alignment with your shoulders. Engage your belly to support your lower back and engage the postural muscles between your shoulders to support your upper body, neck, and head. Maintain a soft gaze as you focus your attention on your breath. Feel your chest expand and your spine lengthen with each inhalation. Use your Inner Core for support as you exhale and release tension from your body and mind. Stay for 10-12 breaths, cultivating a sense of grounding and inner balance.

Standing Side Bend

Standing sideways on your mat, place your feet slightly wider than hip-width apart. Create a Mountain Pose alignment in your body, stabilizing your pelvis by drawing in your abdominals.

(a) As you inhale, reach your right hand out to the side and turn your palm upward. Without pivoting your hips, reach up overhead just past center until you feel a stretch along the right side of your torso. As you exhale, press your right arm down and turn your head to the left. Repeat the movement 3 times, feeling the stretch above your waist.

(b) Then, once again come into the side bend as you inhale. This time, stay in the side bend and exhale, bending your elbow in a lat-bar pull configuration, pulling down with the muscles inside your shoulder blade and twisting your chest to the right. Simultaneously, release your head in the opposite direction to look down towards your left foot. This creates a nice stretch for your neck. Repeat this movement. 3 times, turning your head to center as you inhale and looking down towards your left foot as you breathe out. Then, on inhalation lift up and return back to **Mountain Pose**. Pause and feel. Take the **Standing Side Bend** on your second side. *Remember to stabilize your lower back by engaging your abdominal core.*

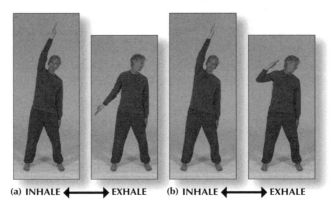

(a) INHALE ←——→ EXHALE   (b) INHALE ←——→ EXHALE

Standing Forward Bend

Stand on your mat in **Mountain Pose** and check your alignment. Inhale in this position to lengthen your spine. As you exhale, bend your knees slightly and fold forward, while maintaining a straight spine. Once you stretch down half-way towards the floor allow your back to round. Slide your hands down your legs for a comfortable stretch and let your head completely go. As you inhale, press into your legs and lift up as if coming out of **Chair Pose**—legs strong, shoulders rolled back, chest lifted. Repeat 4 times and then stay in the **Forward Bend** for 3-4 breaths to deepen the stretch on the back of your body. Come up as you inhale, engaging your back muscles and your abdominals to provide good postural support for your back. If your back feels strained with your hands resting on your legs, place your hands on the seat of the chair or on the bolster for support.

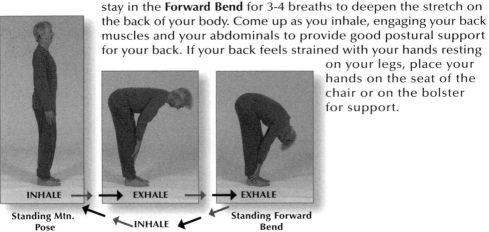

INHALE →   → EXHALE →   → EXHALE

Standing Mtn.   ↖INHALE ←   ← Standing Forward
Pose   Bend

Kneeling Side Bend

Stand on your knees with a blanket for padding. Turn your right leg out to the side, rotating out 90 degrees, positioning your right heel in line with your left knee. Your pelvis is in an open position. Bring your right forearm to rest on your right thigh. Make this arm active, like a brace, imagine you had a basketball under your right rib-cage keeping the whole right side engaged so it doesn't collapse onto your thigh.

(a) Turn your left arm out and as you inhale sweep your left arm up and overhead alongside your ear. As you exhale, sweep your left arm back down by your side and turn your head opposite looking towards your right foot (*as you did in the* **Standing Side-Bend**) Keep your chest lifted at all times. Repeat this movement 3 times; turning your head to the center as you inhale, and looking down to the right as you exhale.

(b) Then, take the lat-bar pull variation (*as in the* **Standing Side Bend**), bending your elbow as you exhale, pulling back and twisting your chest to the left, head turned to the right, stretching your neck. Repeat 3 times. To come out of the pose, lift up with your inhalation breath, pressing through your legs and reaching up with your left arm back to center. Stand on both knees, pause and feel before taking the **Kneeling Side Bend** on your second side.

> If you are unable to kneel, please use the seated variation of the Side Bend. For a full description of Seated Side Bend, see pg. 66.

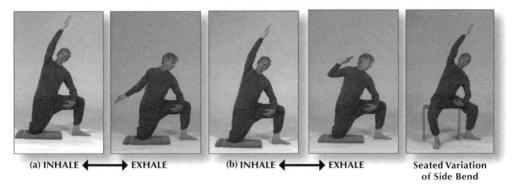

(a) INHALE ⟷ EXHALE   (b) INHALE ⟷ EXHALE   Seated Variation
of Side Bend

Wheel Pose — *Progressive Exhale*

Come onto your hands and knees and place a blanket under your knees for padding. Position your hands shoulder-width apart, directly below your shoulders, and place your knees hip-distance apart, directly below your hips. With your inhalation, lift your tailbone, head, and chest. As you exhale, engage your belly and stretch your hips back to your heels, counting your exhale in one second intervals for 4 counts. Repeat. Lengthen your exhalation to 6 counts and repeat the movement for 2 breath cycles. Then lengthen your exhalation to 8 counts and repeat the movement again for two breath cycles. Rest in **Child's Pose**.

> If you have a knee condition that prohibits you from kneeling, please do the seated, chair variation. For a full description of Seated Wheel, see pg. 64.

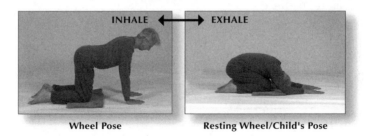

INHALE ⟷ EXHALE

Wheel Pose   Resting Wheel/Child's Pose

The Essential Low Back Program   59

Cobra — *Swimmer's Variation*

Come onto your belly with hands resting just outside your shoulders, forearms on the floor, elbows by your ribs. Begin with your feet hip-width apart. Let your feet stretch back, tops of your feet on the floor. Inhale and lift your chest and your legs, straddling your legs wide apart. Pause. Exhale and squeeze your thighs together, keeping your chest and legs lifted. Release and relax your chest and legs to the floor. Take a breath in the resting position, then repeat the lift, straddle and squeeze movement for a total of 6 cycles. As you feel strong enough, try 2 or 3 repetitions of the straddle and squeeze movement in a row without resting. *Build strength gradually with this posture. Don't push.*

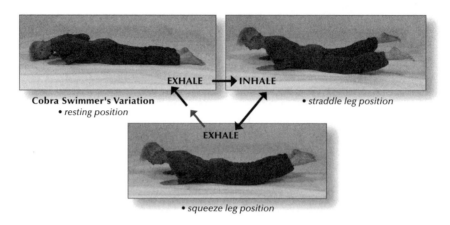

Cobra Swimmer's Variation
• *resting position*
EXHALE ➝ INHALE
• *straddle leg position*
EXHALE
• *squeeze leg position*

Extended Leg Pose — *Straddle Leg Variation*

(a) Lie on your back and place a blanket under your neck if you need the support to keep your neck relaxed. Bend your knees into your chest and place your hands behind the backs of your knees. Exhale in this position. On the inhale, extend your legs so your heels press up towards the ceiling. Repeat 3 times.

(b) On your next inhale, extend your legs fully and straddle them wide, keeping your lower back pressing firmly into the floor. Hands press into your inner thighs to keep the legs very active. As you exhale, slowly squeeze your thighs together. Repeat this movement 3 times, progressively slowing the exhalation breath and movement. *(Keep your knees slightly flexed, to ensure your lower back rests safely on the floor).*

(c) When finished exhale and fold your knees into your chest, then rest your feet on the floor. Pause and feel the effect of the pose.

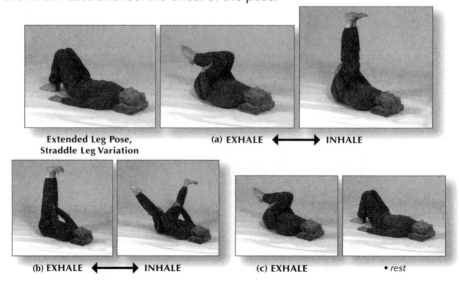

Extended Leg Pose,
Straddle Leg Variation
(a) EXHALE ⟷ INHALE
(b) EXHALE ⟷ INHALE
(c) EXHALE
• *rest*

Lying Twist

Lie on your back and place your feet on the floor. Lift your right foot up and cross your right knee over your left. Spread your arms out into a soft T-shape. As you exhale, draw your belly in and twist to the left, keeping your left foot on the floor and using the support of your left leg to monitor how deeply you move into the twist. Allow your head to turn to the right. Inhale, and return to center. Repeat this movement 3 times, twisting as you exhale, and return to the center as you inhale. As you exhale the fourth time, stay in the twist for 3 breaths. Come out of the twist as you inhale and perform the **Knees to Chest Pose** before repeating the **Lying Twist** sequence on your other side.

*Place a blanket or bolster under your knees if there's any strain on your lower back. If your low back or sacrum feel strained **at all** with this movement, please practice the **Butterfly Pose** instead.*

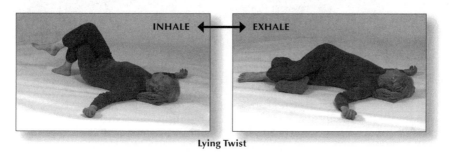

Lying Twist

Butterfly Pose – *2-Part Exhalation Variation*

Turn the soles of your feet to meet one another, allowing your hips to open. Inhale and expand your breath from the chest to belly. As you exhale, slowly squeeze your thighs together, engaging your belly and the muscles of your upper legs, pressing your lower back into the floor. Inhale and open your legs. Exhale slowly and consciously, stabilizing your pelvic girdle. Repeat this movement 6 times. Next, divide the exhalation movement and breath into two equal parts, like this: First, close your thighs halfway and exhale half the breath. Pause. Then continue to breathe out and bring your thighs together. Repeat for another 6 breath cycles keeping the exhalation movement slow and conscious and keeping all pelvic muscles engaged.

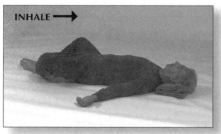

(a) **Butterfly Pose**

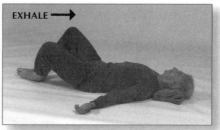

(b) • *Exhale, half way pause*

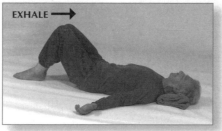

(c) • *exhale all the way*

Knee to Chest Pose

Lie on your back and draw both knees up until you can place one hand on each knee. As you exhale, fold your knees into your chest, stretching your low back. As you inhale, release your knees back until they are arm's length away from you *(feet stay off the floor)*. Repeat 6 times, progressively slowing the exhaled breath and movement.

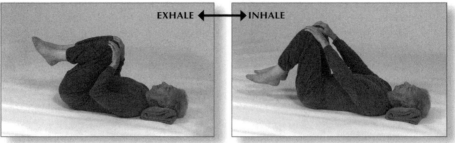

Knee to Chest Pose

Relaxation Pose

Arrange yourself comfortably and consciously on the floor. Place the bolster or chair under your knees so your low back can relax in a neutral position. Evenly spread your body across the floor, so you feel balanced right to left. Allow your whole body to rest. Relax your breath, keeping your mind focused on the movement of the breath and the gentle release of muscular tension. Remain in this position for 3-5 minutes.

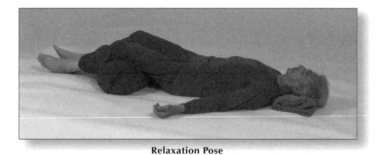

Relaxation Pose

Seated Pranayama/Deep Yoga Breathing

Come into a **Seated Mountain Pose**, either in a chair or in a simple cross-legged position on the floor. Sit comfortably using a blanket or bolster under your sitbones so that you are able to hold your spine erect without great effort. Keeping your focus on your breath, expand your chest as you inhale. As you exhale, draw your belly in from your pubic bone to your navel, then continue to draw in from your navel to your solar plexus, flattening your lumbar curve as you press the breath out of your body.

Progressively lengthen your exhalation to 8 counts. Take several breath cycles to achieve this, keeping the breath long and smooth and the inhalation free and open. Once you've exhaled to the count of 8, divide the breath into two parts: For the first part, breathe out for 4 counts, drawing in from your lower abdominals *(pubic bone to navel)*. Pause. For the second part, breathe out for 4 counts, engaging your upper abdominals *(navel to solar plexus)*. Inhale and relax your belly as you expand from the top down. Repeat this 2-part exhale for 12 breath cycles. When you've completed your breathing practice, relax and breathe naturally. Stay for another 6-12 breaths, experiencing the effects of your practice.

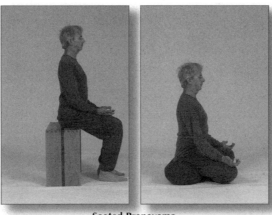

Seated Pranayama

LIFE REFLECTIONS:

What does it feel like when my body,
heart and mind are in alignment?

How much of my life do I live with that sense of connectivity?

~

What does it mean to be in right relationship with my body?
How can I care for my body with tenderness and love?

~

There's nowhere to go, nothing to do, no one to be,
other than myself, here, experiencing this moment just as it is.

SEATED VARIATIONS OF KNEELING POSTURES

Seated Wheel Pose

Begin all of the **Seated Wheel Pose Variations** in this way. Come to a **Seated Mountain Pose** at the edge of the chair with your hips well-supported with a blanket, so your hips are slightly higher than your knees. Align your feet and knees hip width-apart and rest your hands on your thighs.

As you inhale, lift your tailbone and extend your head and chest, drawing your shoulders down away from your ears, forming a back bend or "smile" position. As you exhale, engage your belly, fold forward, tucking your tailbone under, allowing your hands to slide down your legs, forming a domed or rounded back. Feel the stretch.

Follow the specific breathing instructions given in the regular practice you are working on.

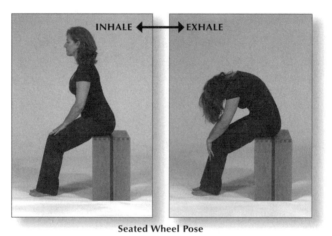

Seated Wheel Pose

Seated Child's Pose

Exhale and release into the forward bend as you do with **Seated Wheel Pose**. Let your head and neck hang freely. Relax your arms completely. If your belly feels compressed at all, widen your legs so there's more room to comfortably release forward. Stay for 6 breaths. To come up, use your legs, abdominals and spine to support you, let your hands slide up your legs.

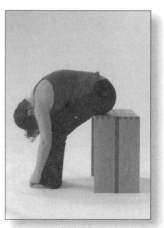

Seated Child's Pose

Seated Thunderbolt Pose

Come to a **Seated Mountain Pose** at the edge of the chair with your hips well-supported with a blanket, so your hips are slightly higher than your knees. Align your feet and knees hip-width apart and rest your hands on your lower back. As you inhale, raise both arms in front of you and then overhead, lengthening your spine. As you exhale, draw your abdominals in and bend forward, sweeping your arms out to the sides and resting the back of the hands to your lower back. Release your head and neck. Once again, on inhalation, extend your spine, reaching out through your arms, lifting your chest. Repeat the movement 6 times. Keep your feet well-grounded and release your neck as you fold forward to avoid tension.

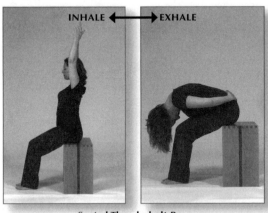

INHALE ← → EXHALE

Seated Thunderbolt Pose

Seated Lunge *(need a bolster or firm pillow to rest the back knee)*

Sit sideways on a chair with only your right buttock on the chair. Place a bolster or firm pillow under your left knee for support and relax your knee into it. Position yourself so that your right buttock is well-supported, your right shin perpendicular to the floor, and your right foot firmly planted. Rest your left foot topside down so your foot is pointing straight back. Shift your left leg back until you feel a deep stretch on the front on the left thigh and hip. Lift your chest slightly, resting your hands on your right thigh. Continue to drop into the stretch on your left hip and groin. Support your lower back by drawing your abdominals in. Keep your breath moving steadily as you stay in the position, 3-4 breaths. Then, as you inhale, lean slightly forward and reach up with your left arm to increase the stretch on the left side. As you exhale, press your arm forward and down. Repeat this arm movement 3 times, then stay and hold the stretch with your left arm up for 3 more breaths. Release out of the stretch, bring your left leg forward. Sit in **Seated Mountain Pose**. Pause and feel the effect of the posture. Repeat the **Seated Lunge** sequence on the other side with your right leg back and your right arm raised.

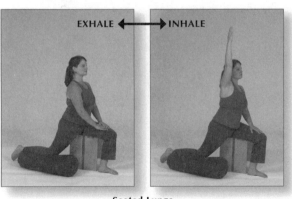

EXHALE ← → INHALE

Seated Lunge

Seated Side Bend

Position yourself on the chair in a wide-legged **Mountain Pose** with your hips turned out and pelvis open. Bring your right forearm or hand to rest on your right thigh. Press into this arm holding it firm, like a brace, ensuring that the whole right side of your body is lifted and not collapsed or sagging. Turn your left arm out and as you inhale sweep your left arm up and overhead alongside your ear. Drop your inner shoulders down, so there is space between your shoulders and your ear. As you exhale, sweep your left arm back down by your side and turn your head to look to the right, towards your right foot. Keep your chest lifted at all times. Repeat this movement 3 times, turning your head center as you inhale, and looking down to your right foot as you exhale. Feel the stretch on the left side of your neck as you turn right and sweep your left arm down. Then, take the lat-bar pull variation: Staying in the side bend, on inhale reach your left arm overhead, as you exhale bend your elbow and pull back from your shoulder blade, twisting your chest to the left. Continue to turn your head to look down to your right on exhale. Repeat 3 times. To come out of the pose, extend out through both arms as you inhale, pressing down into your legs and lifting your spine back to center. Sit in **Mountain Pose**, arms relaxed. Pause and feel the effect of the posture before taking the **Seated Side Bend** on the other side.

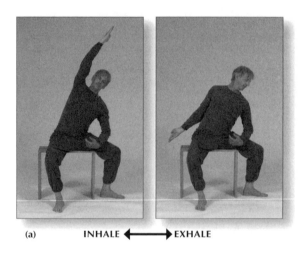

(a)　　INHALE ◄————► EXHALE

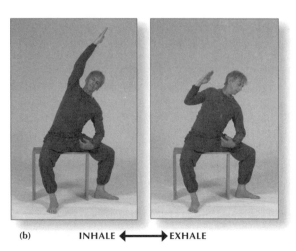

(b)　　INHALE ◄————► EXHALE

References and Resource Material

Benjamin, Ben with Borden, Gail, (1984), *Listen to Your Pain,* New York. Penguin Books.

Desikachar, T.K.V., (1995), *The Heart of Yoga,* Rochester, VT. Inner Traditions International.

Devi, Nischala Joy, (2000), *The Healing Path of Yoga,* New York. Three Rivers Press.

Farhi, Donna, (1986), *The Breathing Book,* New York. Owl Books.

Farhi, Donna, (2003) *Bringing Yoga to Life,* New York. Harper-Collins.

Kraftsow, Gary, (1999), *Yoga for Wellness,* New York. Penguin Books.

Lasater, Judith, (2000), *Living Your Yoga,* Berkeley, CA. Rodmell Press

Lasater, Judith, (1995), *Relax and Renew,* Berkeley, CA. Rodmell Press

Myers, Thomas, (2004), *Anatomy Trains,* Elsevier Limited, China.

Mohan, A.G., (1993),*Yoga for Body, Breath and Mind,* Portland OR. Rudra Press.

Mohan, A.G. and Indra, (2004), *Yoga Therapy,* Shambhala Publications, Boston, MA.

Myss, Caroline, (1996), *Anatomy of Spirit,* New York. Three Rivers Press.

Sarno, John E., M.D., (1991), *Healing Back Pain,* New York. Warner Books.

Sapolsky, Robert, M., (1998), *Why Zebras Don't Get Ulcers,* New York. Henry Holt, & Co. L.L.C.

Schatz, Mary Pullig, (1992), *Back Care Basics,* Berkeley, Rodmell Press.

Sherman KJ, Cherkin DC, Erro J, Miglioretti DL, Deyo RA. *Comparing yoga, exercise, and a self-care book for chronic low back pain: a randomized, controlled trial.* Ann Intern Med. 2005;143:849-56.

A special thanks to Matthew J. Taylor, PT, PhD, RYT for sharing his unpublished dissertation with me: Taylor, MJ (2005) *Re-membering Our Back Pain.*

ROBIN ROTHENBERG

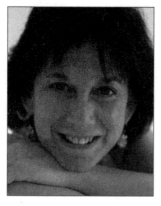

Robin Rothenberg began her own yoga journey as a way to recoup her health and alleviate lower back strain post child-birth. It was the healing capacity of yoga that inspired her to become a teacher, so she could share her experience in a way that would inspire others to heal themselves. Certified in both the *Iyengar* and *Viniyoga* traditions and an AVI Certified Yoga Therapist, she has been teaching yoga for over 20 years. Robin is the owner of **The Yoga Barn**, a thriving studio in Issaquah, Washington, offering more than 40 classes a week for all levels, and featuring a Therapeutic Yoga Program with individual and group classes. (www.yogabarn.com)

Robin is recognized by colleagues as a highly skilled yoga therapist and trains teachers at the Yoga Alliance 500-hour level. Robin sits on the Advisory Board for the International Association of Yoga Therapists (IAYT). She is also an instructor and Advisory Committee Member for Mount Royal College's Yoga Therapy Program in Calgary, which will launch in August, 2008. Robin has presented on low back pain at the IAYT Symposiums for 2007 and 2008. She also presented on "Yoga for Anxiety" at the NAMA (National Ayurvedic Medical Association) conference in 2007.

Robin created the **Pacific Institute of Yoga Therapy** to help establish yoga therapy as a healing profession. She now offers **The Essential Low Back Program: Teacher Training Intensive**, to teach registered instructors how to adapt practices specifically for students with lower back pain. She also offers annual teachers' retreats, as well as open retreats each year in wonderful settings such as Guatemala, Mexico and Costa Rica.

For more information about Robin's trainings and retreats, or to host Robin in your area, visit: **www.piyogatherapy.com** or e-mail: **info@piyogatherapy.com**

ORDER FORM

To order additional copies of **The Essential Low Back Program: Relieve Pain & Restore Health**, use one of the following methods:

1) Telephone Call **1-800-BOOK LOG (1-800-266-5564) Toll Free**. Have your credit card ready.

2) Internet: Go to **www.piyogatherapy.com** and follow the ordering instructions

3) Postal Orders: Send a copy of this page with a check to: **Pacific Institute of Yoga Therapy**, c/o Atlas Books, 30 Amberwood Parkway, Ashland, OH 44805

NO OF COPIES	PRICE	TOTAL
The Essential Low Back Program: Relieve Pain & Restore Health _____	$49. 95	_____
Shipping UPS Ground: $7.00 plus $1.00 per additional item (Allow 7-10 days for delivery)		_____
Your Local Sales Tax, where applicable		_____
	Total $	_____